TEASE ME, PLEASE ME, WHIP ME, BEAT ME

By Mistress G

Mistress G

Published by
Chipmunkapublishing
PO Box 6872
Brentwood
Essex CM13 1ZT
United Kingdom

http://www.chipmunkapublishing.com

Edited by Kimberley Bishop

TEASE ME, PLEASE ME, WHIP ME, BEAT ME

'I know something better than sex', he said. That's nice said I nonchalantly.

That's me all over, let them work at it, he will tell me if he wants to and he is trying hard to make me interested. He had been trying to entertain me with stories of his time in Thailand, all sexually explicit.

I knew he had an interest in BDSM, he was always talking of his escapades.... how he would take a girl out to the forest and tie her to a tree and flog her, tie her up, put her naked in the boot of his car and drive to an abandoned barn, bundle her out and leave her there, naked and anticipating.

Not knowing what was to come. That he would come back with several men and watch them fuck her, was her fantasy, would he fulfil it....

'She was creaming herself thinking of what was to come', he said. She was shivering with cold and anticipation....

He was trying to build me up to his way of thinking, he had been doing it for years, and he could see something in me that I couldn't see myself. I had always seen myself as a person who tried to please everyone, a bit forthright and liking things my own way and ruling my kids with looks and a metaphorical iron rod.

In the end, he got himself so wound up that he had to tell me why he had come to visit.

My friend, who I knew of, as a Dominant wanted me to Dominate him. Jeez what the hell do I do? He gave me half an hour to digest this. My poor little unimaginative mind was whirling, Domination. DOMINATION. Oh My God...

He was getting excited at the prospect of me playing with him, It was a hot day, so I told him he should go to the bathroom and strip, he would be bathing me, drying me then dressing me.

I wasn't used to these things happening to me so I was putting on a brave front, quaking in my boots really. My instincts telling me that this wasn't what he wanted, but I hadn't a clue what he did want. When we went into the bedroom, him with a submissive stance, well nearly, he was putting on a half hearted attempt, making it hard for me to read him, not that I knew what I was looking for.

He then opened his Aladdin's cave, his bag, and showed me the goodies within... What on earth was I to do with deep heat? That stuff hurts like hell where am I to put that... where it won't hurt him too much. Poor naive me, mistake number one, I didn't apply it.

Then there were things that looked like they would really hurt, 'those go on your nipples...really? Ouch.
You don't honestly want me to hit you with this do you?'
God I was so stupid, I hadn't got my head around any of the concept of BDSM...

TEASE ME, PLEASE ME, WHIP ME, BEAT ME

This chap made me feel very uncomfortable, I was out of my comfort zone, he was not able to teach me, coach me, help me in any way. Though in the future, it seems his approach to introducing me to this way of life worked. He continued to be very unhelpful when I went to him time and time again to learn more. He said it had to come from within, to be natural. But just what was it I had to do? To feel?

At first he let me watch some videos, then let me take some home, they looked amateur and silly, women inflicting pain on men, they weren't enjoying what they were doing, so why do it, dead pan faces, then screaming and shouting at their clients, why?
I could never do that, and to this day never have.

Still he wouldn't tell me anything about the mentality of the Scene, I would have to work it out for myself. I'm really not sure why I pursued this way of life, as I thought at the time it went against everything I believed in. But the longer I play with people the more I understand. Giving them a release from thinking, being mindless for a while, a release from responsibility.

I get a lot of pleasure from My work, I have learned...or was it always there? To read people, to make a session flow, to know what they want and to give it to them. But though I have gone back and played with My friend once, I could never go there again, I would not get any satisfaction from him, I need to feed from My submissives enjoyment, and he shows none, he is too busy trying to direct the scenario, getting no pleasure as he won't give into the enjoyment...

CHAPTER ONE

My father was a very gentle man. Not a forward thinking man, more live for the moment, as I recollect not Dominant or submissive, but then at that time I wouldn't know what that was even if it had bent down and bit Me on the bum.

He was a Padre in the forces, a hard job as the war was on. In every aspect of his life he drew people to him, they trusted him and felt able to take advantage of him. He was often the brunt of jokes, which he was happy to regale. I remember he was once asked if he wanted a trip in an aircraft, game for anything My father jumped at the chance. Suited and booted with the obligatory packet of fags in his pocket he set off. He wasn't enjoying the trip much, in those days they didn't have the comforts of today's planes, but not one to show these things he was laughing and joking and generally taking his mind off the trip. Deciding that things were getting out of control and he needed to calm his nerves he reached for his cigarettes, the pilot passed a knowing look across to his mate, who grinned and gave the thumbs up. My father thinking they were asking if he was OK, nodded and grinned, fishing a cigarette from the packet, he offered them around, rooting in his pockets he managed to find a packet of matches, so intent was he on finding the matches that he hadn't noticed that the plane was descending, and starting to loop the loop. In his fumbling and the angle of the plane plus the force of the plane dropping, he dropped the matches. Bent down to pick them up and couldn't get back up again, try as he might to get up he was stuck there, They thought it great fun, but he was getting greener and greener, he didn't know how long he was bent over for but it felt like a lifetime and in the end he brought up his lunch, though he didn't go into much detail on that, I do know that the pilots found it highly entertaining and when they returned to the ground the story went round the base like wildfire. My father was the brunt of much joshing for a while after, but as was his way, he turned it to his advantage, he had a great rapport with the lads and they always came to him with their problems and the father I knew must have sent them away feeling a lot happier.

My father met My mother near the end of the war. Now that must have been a happy time, end of war parties, though rationing was still in force. All would have been well except that My father was already married...He had a wife and two children. He had big decisions to make. It broke his heart to leave the children and he was to find out that his ex wife would not allow contact if he left.

My father, a trusting soul, not able to see any wrong in anyone, very naive, went into partnership with a friend, a dry cleaning business.
He was well and truly taken to the cleaners. Fleeced of his savings
We moved to a little village in Somerset where My very intelligent father went to work in a plastics factory. He hated the work and losing a finger to a

hungry cutting machine was the last straw, he decided that poverty while he took a course to be a teacher was the only option. As a learned man, university educated, he didn't need the years of training, which was lucky for us as we only saw him at weekends.

For a middle-aged man to take a career change so late in life, with a family to support was a hard choice to make. Going into the work at a single persons wage was hard, but My mother coped, as everyone else has had to in those days. We all had big gardens and the farmers seemed to like our family so pheasants and rabbits found their way to our door to supplement the vegetables.

My fathers motor bike, which was the cheapest way for him to travel was replaced by a bubble car, a source of amusement for all, as eccentric as My father with its front lifting door, and the steering wheel perched in the middle of it. It was great fun to go for a drive if I was lucky enough. It did not fit a family of five though. Then joy of joys, eventually we could all go out in a car together. My father bought an estate car. It had wood panelling down the sides. My pride of place was right at the back. Ballast probably as I wasn't the lightest of little girls. A trip to the largest of towns meant all of us chugging up the hills, willing the car to make it, all of us urging the car on, physically moving the car, with our bodies rocking back and forth.

When I was about nine we moved from our lovely house next to the local church. My father was the organ player, and my brother; sister and myself were in the choir. Twice every Sunday and weddings and funerals. As my siblings got older they did not have to go anymore, so that meant sometimes there were only two in the choir. myself and another girl. She couldn't hold a note and her and I used to belt out the hymns, competing with each other to be the loudest. My father never uttered a word about the obvious fools we were making of each other. But we must have been the laughing stock of the village.

E Stem

I have a voice activated E Stem, I love using it on new clients, I can have them connected to it and administer the shocks, leave it a while and do something else, then as I'm talking to them, laugh, I laugh a lot while I'm working, because I enjoy it so. My laugh sets the box off, it's just the right pitch to send shock waves through the system and they jump at the unexpectedness off it. No I can't shatter a crystal glass with My shrieks, it's a low pitch.

We moved into a big Manse house, it hadn't been lived in for years. My father spent many long nights clearing the brambles and nettles from around the place, as you couldn't reach the front door, then making the place habitable. It was a couple of years before the place was ready to move into.

Nettles and Switches

Seeing the verges covered with nettles, I decided to cut a bunch I only stung Myself once. I had great plans for it.

My new slave is a masochist. I can do anything to him, he works all the harder for Me, with a better frame of mind if I beat him, he has been without his fix for so long he is very grateful and adoring for every little crumb I bestow on him.
The nettles wrapped in fabric so I wouldn't get stung, were applied to his bared back, he was stripped, as his back wasn't the only place I was going to flog.
his arms spread wide, resting on My new medieval chest, legs spread, and he was waiting with trepidation. he had not seen what was coming, wrapped up in the thought of what he might receive, he had not thought to tell Me that he was allergic to the nettles he had seen resting, ready for use on My freezer.

After three swipes on his back reality hit him and he had a predicament, he felt it necessary to tell Me of his allergy, but it was going against My wishes, but knowing I would have his safety at the forefront of everything, he spoke up, and was sent packing to get some tablets to alleviate the stings. We now have a stock for future mishaps.

I think he knows the joys that were denied him when he reached his home that night. Humm, now what gives that sort of pain and itching, I must set My mind to that.

CHAPTER TWO

A walk in the forest is interesting. One very cold day I decided that I wanted some fresh air as I was bored, so I donned My Harley Davidson boots that had been lovingly polished by slave, lots of warm clothes on and rope tucked in My pocket.
Off Wwe set. I told slave to drive into the heart of the forest. Wwe found a nice spot near a dog-walking trail. Wwe looked at some birds and had a little walk, on finding a likely tree I told him to strip. he started to shiver as I tied him to the tree, arms hugging the tree, legs spread wide. Then I put a blindfold on him. he could hear Me rustling about, and twigs snapping, I had found a nice branch and was making it to My liking, the right size and shape. It was just right, not too smooth.
Stepping up to him, he knew what was coming, I raised the switch and brought it down on his back, leaving a nice welt, liking the sight of that, I gave him a few more, until his back was covered, he was shivering well by the time I had finished so I took pity on him and let him lose.

Seeing how cold he was, I decided I had better warm him up, as I needed the loo, I told him to squat under Me and I gave him a drink. But as he was so cold and perched at a funny angle not much went into his mouth so I peed over him instead, warming him that way. When I finished I told him to get dressed. Wwe then trotted off back to the car, him shivering damply, Me happy with My work and not bored any more. Neither was he when he got home, as he had to clean My boots again, till they were pristine.

With the house came a church, complete with graveyard and the option for the last Moravian dwellers to be buried there. They were thin on the ground, but we did have the occasional burial there. A school, out buildings and some land. The land was rented out to a farmer who every year used to spread chicken manure. Oh the smell...It made your eyes water and made it difficult to breath, but the grass grew well.

The night of the day we moved in, the local farmers gave us a welcoming present. They had set rook scarers in the trees surrounding our grounds, the first one had us all jumping out of bed, thinking the war had broken out again, My father went out to investigate but could not find anything. Off to bed we all went again, only to be roused every half an hour through the night by these immensely noisy pest scarers.
It was a great honour for us that the farmers thought enough of us to pull this prank

My father taught the remedials as they were then called, but as he never taught them, just told them stories, they thought he was the best thing since sliced bread, mind I don't think sliced bread was popular then, I don't remember seeing it about till later, we had to slice our own.

These children went on to take exams that normally would have been denied them, I faired worse than them, I didn't take any. These tamed children took such a liking to My father that the biggest meanest bully and his cronies used to cycle five miles to help My father with our vast garden.

When My father died, we found that My mother had to move out of the family home because My father hadn't paid a peppercorn rent to My aunt, his sister,

The only contact I had with My half siblings was at My father's funeral, I think he might have seen them once or twice when they were grown up. They kept in touch with My father's side of the family though, as I was to find out at My aunts funeral.

My aunt was a very bossy woman, wanted things her own way. She organized everyone, got up everyone's noses. She lived in a little village and tried to run it. She was a member of the church where everything needed to be done her way, I think the fact she and her husband weren't short of a bob or two might have helped a little in the beginning but you can only tolerate such behaviour for so long.

My Mother found out that My aunt had died, not many months after her husband. We went to the funeral. There weren't many in the church, they took our names before we went in. We sat at the back where I discovered a cat had decided to put its mark on My cushion. It was a foul smell and I had to spend the rest of the day stinking to high heaven and hoping no one else could smell it.

We didn't know anyone, but went back to her house afterwards and found that she only had acquaintances, no one really close to her.
They seemed quite excited that I was there and asked Me to leave My address and asked for that of My brother as well. I clicked on straight away and had to tell them that it wasn't Me they wanted but My fathers first daughter, who's name was a shortened version of Mine. I was the only blood relative there and My mother was next closest kin. Of course we weren't recognized in the will, as My father had blotted his copybook, by marrying My mother.

Domination

A lot of people like to be bossed about, being told what to do, not thinking for themselves, to be scalded for not doing things right. Some like to be shouted at and verbally abused. Put down and made to feel inferior, to be kicked and hit as a form of humiliation.

If you people watch, when you next go shopping, how often do you see one partner, walking behind another, carrying all the bags and being scolded for one reason or another. The hen pecked husband...The put upon wife.... People not in the scene, feel sorry for them, but they are in their element, exactly where they want to be. Enjoying every minute.

I don't shout and holler I control with looks and actions, quietly issuing orders either in their faces or whispering in their ears. I'm not very verbal.

CHAPTER THREE

I was born In Peacehaven, Sussex the third child of my parents. Helped into this world by a midwife whose name I bear as my parents hadn't chosen one for me. My grandmother was there as well, to help tend us all, right down to the fact of bringing some heating as it was a cold and frosty day that I chose to arrive, all huddled into the only room with heat. I think it should have been a memorable day, but my grandmother could never remember the date,

I loved my grandma; she was a cantankerous old dear and my best friend. I could escape to her when things were bad for me and she was the person who got me my first bra, the one to cover my gnat bites, I was the envy of the bouncy girls who's parents would not admit their little girls were growing up.

She lived to be a hundred, cursing every day past the age of eighty; I brought her to live near me so I could put a little sunshine into her life. The rest home was a nice enough place, some caring people, and me popping in with her favourite grandson helped. Though I do know that she probably had a moan about us when we left. Moaning seemed to be her favourite pastime, nothing was ever right but if it kept her happy, we were happy to let her do it.

TEASE ME, PLEASE ME, WHIP ME, BEAT ME

She was a feisty old bird and the source of many a story and I tried to glean as much information from her before she died. I feel sorry that I didn't record her tales on tape. Born in 1899, that seems very strange, as we are now in year 2007, a very long time ago.

She saw five great great grandchildren born but missed the only girl among them. A girl who is the spitting image of her in looks.

Hands on hips, legs spread in stance, very red face. Very indignant that I'm being queried, I'm not wrong, how could I be wrong, I'm never wrong.... I have been sent back to my chair to solve the problem, why should I do it again, I have done it three times already, I have counted, recounted and counted yet again, two and two do make five, they do! I can't make it anything else.

My teacher in nursery class had been patient with me at first, faced with a little fireball, standing her ground but without the vocabulary to argue back, all I can shout is 'I'm right' she starts to shout back but recovers her composure realising that it's only a five year old she is dealing with. Exasperated she sits me down towering above me, all five foot nothing of her; she patiently goes through the problem with me.
I can't believe it, how do I back down from this, I have been proved wrong. How did that happen? I'm thinking hard, the angry red indignant face is now blushing and rather shamed faced, I pull my

shoulders back and say 'well, if you want it to be four, I will let you.' I then receive the dressing down of my life, as I'm shrivelling inside, my exterior bristling, my back getting straighter and straighter.... I admit defeat...but not enough so, because I am told to apologise.... APOLOGISE.... no way.
Start of another argument, Both of us, not going to budge, ending with me losing my playtime as I'm stood in the corner, hands on head. Feeling very sorry for myself and as there's no one around to hear, I finally give in, and mumble I'm sorry. That was the start of my rebellious time at school. Mind I tried to keep myself to myself most of the time, plus I think wanting things my own way might have put some of the children off being around me.

School Room

Sitting at their desks, dressed in uniform, with schoolbooks, rulers and pens at the ready, the pupils waiting for the lesson to begin. Teacher dressed in mortar and coat, cane in hand, slapping it against thigh, letting the pupils know what is to come if they misbehave.

Lots of giggling, fighting and paper throwing. Anything to get noticed. Not getting questions right, and fidgeting.

jim throws a ball of paper, which misses target or does it? It hits Teacher. Get to the front of class, bend over, touch your toes, six of the best. jim receives the stripes, yelping, then rises when told and is sent back to his desk, rubbing his bottom, happy with the result, but looking shamefaced, as all the rest laugh at his misfortune, but thinking of their turn to come.

Sitting in the shade head in hands to block out the sunlight. One little girl, well maybe not so little, I was a chubber. Fighting the nausea, yet another migraine, not the best scholar I found things hard at school. Looking back, perhaps that was my way out of things. No one understood these things. I was the only one in my family to get any illness. Everyone else was as fit as fiddles.

I only lived a hundred yards from the local church school, but had to sit the rest of the day out getting more and more nauseas, till at last I threw up and was sent home to sleep and spend the next 24hrs in bed, not sleeping but saying hello to God every 15mins. Mind it could also have been something I ate that didn't agree with me because after my spell in bed I was fit and raring to go, on top form, not so later in my life, when after these spells I would be washed out. Mind that may have been because with a family to look after you can't take as much time off as you need.

As I got older, I realized that if I wanted a day off from school I could wake up with one, and not go into school with My father, who taught at the secondary school, I went to. It was a day spent in bed though, not that I minded, I always did need a lot of sleep and being an avid reader I expect a lot of time was spent under the covers with a torch instead of sleeping.

As I got older I realized that I was rubbish at English, I couldn't spell, I would spend hours, well a bit of an exaggeration, but the walk to school at least, learning my ten set spellings.

I loved tests, still do, but I wasn't given multiple choice, the headmaster who would walk up and down the lines of us terrified children, well the dunces like me, not the brainiacs, with a plimsoll, hitting the palm of his hand, just to let us know what we would get if we got any wrong.

The line waiting for our bottoms to be hit would be quite long and more often than not, I was in it, shaking in my sensible shoes, dreading my turn. The boys joking and saying it wouldn't hurt, like the big brave men they were, and us girls just shaking and ready to cry as soon as it was our turn, not that that did us any good. Lift up the skirt, and wallop, a cold beating on the bum. To this day I can't spell so it didn't do me a lot of good.

But I did learn that repetition can make things stick in the brain, if only for a little while and I used to spend ages with My children going through their spellings and their times tables.

TEASE ME, PLEASE ME, WHIP ME, BEAT ME

They went to school in an era that didn't teach you your times tables in a parrot fashion, as I learnt mine, so at every opportunity I would reel off whichever they were learning, it didn't do any good as it was always met with lalalalalala and ears blocked with hands.

I remember idyllic summer days, not only did the farmers have milking herds, but also they had apple trees. The fruit looked very appetising, rosy red apples and lots of them, but bite into one and they tasted foul, they screwed up your mouth and eyes. Spitting them out didn't help, as the damage had been done, and the texture was in your screwed up little mouth for a long time. These apples were cider apples.

They nestled in the damp long grass and as a family, we all scrabbled on our hands and knees to pick them up and pop them into buckets. They were never ending and I hated the job. My attention span being limited, I always wanted to be elsewhere, doing more interesting things, but the camaraderie there was good. The village seemed to me to be there in force. I was too young then to be left alone but I was old enough to be of some help. As I got older I managed to escape doing these things. I always hated doing things like that; manual labour was never my forte. Nowadays I don't have to do anything manual that I don't want to. I have a stable of slaves to do these things.

Mistress G

I remember watching the cider being made. A layer of straw, a layer of apples, and so on. Then a top put on and a screw pressing the layers together. Squashing the fruit, the juice trickling into a trough. The screw being turned every so often till all the juice was extracted. Coming to look at the resulting liquid after it had been trickling all night, you would see all manner of dead livestock in the trough. The farmer would fish them out, and barrel up the enhanced flavoured liquid, ready for it to mature into the potent stuff that became the main point of parties I was to hold in later life.

My capacity for this stuff was a thing to behold, as I could out drink all my mates.
On the night of my party, I would trot up to the farm nearest our house, carrying a few gallon containers. Knock on the farmer's door and ask if I could buy some cider. He would take me to the barn, bearing a pint glass, which he would precede to fill from the first barrel. I would try it and give the glass to him so he could have some, all the time talking about its taste and other things related to the drink. Passing this drink and the few more that were drawn between us, I would eventually choose which one I wanted, watch him fill the containers, then pay him a pittance and make my merry way home on wobbly legs, to get things ready for the arrival of my friends.

The parties were held in the church vestry, which was decorated in a haphazard way. There were sofas and tables there. The steps to the pulpit were extra seating and the pulpit itself was a cosy place to cuddle up in. We all got very merry and very silly with loud music, but there weren't many houses around to complain. The next morning it would be left to me to clean up the mess left by everyone. Not that it really mattered, as I was the only one to enter the church, it was my hide out.

Drink and drugs do not mix with BDSM play as they dull the senses. It is dangerous to be playing with some, i.e. caning them when You can't be true with Your aim.

CHAPTER FOUR

I have slaves that can do most of the things I need doing. As one slave leaves, for whatever reason, the latest through ill health...another takes his place. I have found in My life that things happen when they are meant to, slot neatly into place at the right time...that all the things that happen, good and bad, are meant to be. It's all a learning curve that helps to build our character and make us the way we are. If we have the patience to wait, then the things we are waiting for will come when the time is right.

I'm still waiting for a nice sports car and a big house in the country that I can make into a glorified play area, scene friendly, where I can entertain most aspects of the BDSM life. I know it will come one day and until that time I am happy to entertain in the dungeon contained in My house.

One November 5th a local farmer had built a huge bonfire and we all set off for a great display of fireworks and potatoes baked in the embers. The potatoes were always hard, but tasted fantastic, a great treat.
The fireworks were impressive, but the bonfire was the thing that drew me, I love fire... Lighting a bonfire in the garden, I love the challenge of burning a soggy wet mass completely, My neighbours curse Me as I have so many fires. I creep out late at night now, when all their washing

should be in, hard luck if it isn't.... I take some dry stuff to start it with, then stand, transfixed, watching the hot plastic drip onto the wet paper, steam and smoke billowing, the smell of the different materials assaulting My nose. At this time, I look furtively round to see if the neighbours have left their windows open or are peering through them cursing Me for indulging in one of My passions.

The flames leaping and making different shapes and colours as it engulfs each different substance, dodging the smoke, but knowing I am going to need a shower when I come in from playing.

Fire Play

Fire play consists of sensations. It can scare a slave by just the fact of putting heat next to their skin. It is not meant to burn the skin. Most times...I do it in many ways and there are always more ways of doing this. You just need imagination but safety has to be forefront in everything You do. It's mind play as much as anything,

I tie balls up tight, to nice shiny orbs, then light a candle. If the balls are hairy, My slaves don't have these, but some clients do. I then run the candle flame at a distance under the balls and backside, the heat running over the skin, nothing to worry about...then as I get closer, the hair starts to singe and shrivel and the smell assaults their noses and they start to panic. Am I going to burn all the hair off? How will they explain that to their partners, am I going to let the flames get out of control and set them on fire, am I going to burn the skin? I love the fear they are emitting, I feed off their emotions.

When I have burnt as much hair off as I feel like, I then get a razor and proceed to dry shave their crown jewels. The fear that I am going to cut them, nick a vessel is in their mind, I haven't yet, but there is always a first time.... The patch that is left bare is so small, as the skin has been stretched tight, it won't notice when I undo them.

Lighting a cotton tipped taper doused in alcohol is frightening in itself for some and can give an instant buzz. The act of it coming close to their skin, even more so. The flame just brushes the skin, just enough to caress. You make sure all hair, theirs and Yours is well out of the way and no-one is wearing hair spray, an instant fire ball if this catches at worst and singed hair if it just catches, one way to get a new hairstyle.... As the taper heat decreases You can run it over the skin and leave a nice trail, pretty patterns loll.

Standing close to my mother so I wouldn't go too close to the fire, the farmer had just taken some potatoes from it and brought them over for us. My mother was busy talking as the farmer lifted his fork and slammed it into the ground so he had his hands free to deal with the potatoes. My squeal of pain went unnoticed as I was a whingy child, also prone to exaggeration, so when I told her the fork was in my foot, she poo pooed it, but at my constant wails she thought she had better look. Sure enough the fork had gone through my wellie and also my foot and was stuck in the ground, matter of factly, it was pulled out, my sock taken off and my foot inspected. The fork hadn't hit anything nasty on the way in so my foot was given a kiss and the evening continued, food can take a lot of things off your mind....

Yum food

Chocolate sauce, Golden syrup, treacle, custard, cream, oh bliss. To have it smeared all over your body, then rubbed in, the slimy, slippery sweet tasting stuff covering every inch of your body. Being able to lick the stuff from coated skin, rubbing bodies together, mixing substances, getting different textures, different flavours mingling. Tipped over your head your hair flattened to your head, the goo running down your face, beckoning to be licked of. Cream cakes and pies splodged onto the nearest piece of anatomy, the 'splat squidge' sound as it lands and the feel as you push the cake onto flesh, the cream exploding from the sides, scooping it up and throwing it at your partner. No worries about where it lands, as you have no clothes on, abandoned fun, hurting no one, highly erotic. Mind, not good for the figure if indulged in too often, if you, like Me, can't resist eating the play stuff.

My friends were mainly boys, I related with them better, I was a tom boy, climbing trees, getting up to mischief, haring about on my boys bike, doing foolhardy dares.

I remember one time we all took it in turns to see how long we could strangle ourselves with a curtain cord. Guess who won.... I had to top the boys all the time, in more ways than one.

Breath control

There are many ways of doing this and can be very dangerous if taken too far.
You need to know how far to take things, to be able to read the person. Some like to lose consciousness, some like to take it, to just before that time. This can take many forms, some are.... smothering with Your hand or anything that comes to hand.
Holding their nose and clamping Your mouth over theirs, not letting them breath.
Or breathing into their mouths as You breath in through Your nose.
There is strangulation, with hands or cord.
Putting a gas mask on them, and restricting the air control.
Putting a bag over the head and controlling how much air is given.
 Face sitting, where You put your posterior on their face, lifting Your body to allow them to breath. To name just a few.

TEASE ME, PLEASE ME, WHIP ME, BEAT ME

I restrain My client, then start to relax him, scratch and smooth his face, tracing his lips with My fingers. Teasing him by putting My fingers in his mouth, letting him suck them, pushing them down his throat. Then cupping My hand covering his mouth and nose. The covering just impeding his breathing. he holds his breath and when he needs to breath, realizes that he can take in a laboured breath. It's not comfortable, but after a while I get bored that he can breath so I let him take a few breaths to recover, then hold his nose, clamp My mouth over his and hold it there, keeping My position even though his head starts to rock back and forth. I then let him expel the air and clamping mouth over his again, I breathe air into his lungs. Letting him breath, but taking in My air. Letting him recover for a while I stand and watch him, calculating when I am going to hitch My skirt and lower My posterior over his face. I sit on his face, feeling his compliance, as he has no choice in the matter as My size eighteen bottom is smothering him. My stocking-ed thighs either side of his face, I lift a little so he can take a breath, but clamp down again firmly, I feel him try to breath out and leave it a little longer. It's getting a trifle warm between My thighs. Lifting up I allow him to breath. he is very red faced and starting to sweat.

I walk around the bed, looking him in the eye the whole time. Smiling in a knowing way. him wondering what's going to happen next, I reach his feet, run My fingertips up the soles, grab his toes and pull his ankles together. I put one knee on the bed to one side of his legs, the other, to the right side; allow My body to slump forwards, My hands either side of his torso. I start to crawl over his body, his cock twitching as My skirt brushes over it. I sit high on his belly My legs holding his arms to his sides tight and lean over so My face is close to his, just looking in his eyes. Then I push off the bed with My hands and quickly clamp them over his throat. I put pressure on his throat garrotting him, watching his face the whole time, feeling the motions of his body through My legs. Feeling him complacent under My hands, accepting of what is happening. he is able to breath but only just. I sit like that for a while then release, allowing him to regain composure. Then do it again, this time I reposition My body, using his neck as a stabilising point for My hands, I ease Myself over his cock and sit on him, grinding My crutch against him. Then let go. Let him breath.

CHAPTER FIVE

At the age of nineish I made friends with some older girls, wanting to be grown up like they were, I took to smoking. Not at all fazed, my father allowed me to smoke, but I had to spend my own money on the cigarettes, not on sweets, This little tubs was happy to do that, I could smoke in the house too, a novelty that soon wore off though, smoking in the house, not the smoking.

Smoking Fetish

I smoke still, which has its advantages. I have clients that like to see Me smoke for many different reasons.... One being they like to watch the smoke being drawn into the mouth in different ways and also to see the smoke being exhaled, bright red lipstick that is left on the butt is compelling, the lips pursed.
The focal point....
Smoke blown into their faces sometimes, restrained and not able to move their faces away. Two, being forced to smoke, Me taking a drag and blowing it into their open mouth, or clamping My mouth round theirs and forcing the smoke down their throats.
Three, using their mouths as an ashtray and forcing them to swallow it, putting the end out on their tongues or on their teeth, making them eat the end, chewing and swallowing the end result. Four, cigarette play, running a lit cigarette over skin, leaving an ash trail, burning any hair in its

path, around and on the nipples is good. Also over the penis, the head as well as the shaft. Putting a cigarette out on flesh, or leaving it next to the skin to burn it.

The sweets thing wasn't a problem for me. I had other sources, one of them being a farmer friend whose coat tails I had clutched from the age of two. I would follow him everywhere. He was a cantankerous ex bank manager. Retired, he owned two cows who I used to 'help' milk, then take a cupful home to drink. My mother wouldn't touch the stuff because she didn't know if the cows had had the injections to render the milk safe to drink. I loved it. Soo rich and creamy. Not like the watery stuff you get today. He used to make ice cream with the cream, oooh yummy. He always had some milk on the slow burner, allowing the cream to thicken, then he would scrape it off and freeze it, when frozen he would scoop some out with a spoon and put it in a cornet, such a treat, real Cornish ice cream is the closest I have come to the taste of it. He also had an endless supply of sweeties that I took full advantage of.
He also had an angry pig in a sty that I used to annoy by walking on the wall penning him in. This was a precarious business as I didn't have the best of balance and often joined the pig in his pen. I got quite quick at scrambling out. The adrenalin rush was good though.

TEASE ME, PLEASE ME, WHIP ME, BEAT ME

Adrenalin Rush

There are soo many ways to get an adrenalin rush. Just thinking about something that you know is going to happen, gives you an adrenalin rush, it's the good feeling you get, the tingly feeling, the anticipation, the jitters. The extreme end is going into hyperspace, your own headspace. The endorphins kicking in just like a drug, the same feeling as a drug, as addictive as a drug, but the bodies own mechanism. Though these endorphins kick in when a person really hurts themselves, like severing a limb, it doesn't take that much pain, not always any pain, to get a person in that state. It's all to do with relaxing and totally trusting the person you are with. Being totally at ease and enjoying the fact that the person is doing what you need them to do to you. When a person has reached that state of mind, it is possible to keep them there for as long as you want, time has no meaning. A good Top will bring the person out of this state very carefully. After care is given, Chocolate is a good idea or fruit juice, the bottom needs looking after, they are in a delicate state and need time to recover.

When my friend died I was surprised that he left me some money in his will. It was a Godsend, as I hadn't two pennies to rub together. The story of my life I never had any money, but at that time I was feeding my family on the family allowance, My partners money paying the bills. We slept under coats and lived on eggs, bread and chips and anything he could bring home from work. He was a chef but couldn't bring much stuff home.

My clothes were bought with birthday and Christmas money. A pair of jeans a year. Last years being patched with the pair from the year before, no trendy rips in those days.

My farmer friend had a dog, in fact he had a few dogs in succession, they all had the same thing in common and all came to an untimely end, because of this.
My friend hated cars, he had a truck that we used to take to visit his friends every Sunday, taking others lives in his hands as he headed straight into oncoming traffic, till they chickened out, people soon got to know they wouldn't get the better of him and pulled over to let him pass. The high light of the Sunday was stopping off to get some pop, Tizer, and sweets.

The successive dogs were all the same breed and I don't remember them looking any different from each other.
They could hear a car coming up the road from a great distance, at first their ears would prick up, then, on him starting to cuss they would jump up and race from the house, running up to the car, attacking its wheels, barking and snarling, then chase the car for about half a mile before running home to be petted. I think that was their frequent exercise apart from them walking round the village with my friend.

TEASE ME, PLEASE ME, WHIP ME, BEAT ME

Everyone hated those dogs. Dogs are not supposed to kill cats, but my brother had two who were killed by these dogs, which I think prompted my brother to accidentally shoot my friend with his air gun.... Not a fatal shot...But he was so cross that nothing was done about the unruly hounds. The police were involved, but I think he was lucky enough to get away with a telling off.

Puppy play

Sometimes it's nice to be looked after, to be petted and played with, to be given love, to drink, eat from a dog bowl, not be treated badly, just play and be happy. Not have to think, though training can involve chastisement.

Some puppies enjoy the power exchange, and need to be kept in order. As with other D/S relationships. A pup can be bound so he has to stay on all fours, hobbled so he can barely move, hooded or be put in mittens so he can't do human things. Not allowed to talk, they are there to be enjoyed. My puppy loves his cuddles; he sits at My feet and Wwe watch the television. he waits to be told he can drink from his bowl.
When he walks through the door he has his collar put on, he is already wearing his unknown collar, an aftershave that he wears each day as he can't wear his leather collar at work. puppy has a few things he enjoys so in the course of an overnight stay he might do three different roles, depending on My mood.

CHAPTER SIX

As in most villages, well most places really, there lurk perverts. Not the consensual kinky type, of which I am one, but child molesters. I know there were some in my village. Some of my friends and I were prey to them. I wonder how they can spot venerable children, mind if they have had these yearnings all their lives, then they must find it quite easy. These things were never talked about, and as I got older I realised that one of my friends was playing one chap. She was using him to her advantage. That was the first time that I realised that sex can be used as a tool. I didn't know anything about working girls and the great service they provide, or about promiscuous women, my friend was on to a good thing,

She was getting lots of presents and money for, well, not a lot really, Only just underage, she had learnt how to tease and please a man, and reap the reward. I stored that into the back of my mind for future reference, I did use womanly wiles to get my own way but didn't exploit the fact. I was never really in a position to extort money from anyone; most of the people I knew didn't have much themselves.

I love the idea of Sugar Daddies. Everyone gets what they want from the relationship. I love to be taken away to nice hotels. Though I do seem to disgrace Myself.

I like My comfort and am not big on exercise. I like gifts and surprises, but then what girl doesn't. I like holidays and being looked after, materialistically and physically. Some of these things, all if I really wanted, can be done by slaves, but its nice to have one man who can provide it all.

Money slaves/pigs

A few men like to provide for their Dommes. they like to be milked of their money, to be held to ransom, blackmailed into giving over their money, have their finances put at a Dommes disposal. Open their bank account let the Domme take what they want. Make the slave work to provide for their Domme. This can be open to abuse or not as the slave and Domme decide. But the Domme has ultimate control over the slaves spending.

some just like to pay a bill or take their Domme shopping.

The 60s, flower power, peace and love. The pill was getting easier to get, though still hard if you were single.

I was never a hippy though my sister was and I learnt how to make my own flared jeans and walked around bare foot, I still like to walk round the house with no shoes, and kick My heels off at the first opportunity.

The nearest town was five miles away, with hardly any buses. I wasn't going to bike in and nor was I going to walk, so I used to hitch hike, furtively looking over my shoulder in case I was sticking my thumb out to anyone my parents knew. It was dangerous, I had been told enough times, but nothing bad ever happened to me and it saved me a lot of money, though the trips home were a bit hairy because when you have to be home at a certain time and you end up walking most of the way home, your excuses can get a bit lame after a time.

There was a cafe in town that we used to hang out at. Given the chance I would go there in the school lunchtimes and eat a plate of chips and try hard to look cool. This rotund teenager in ill-fitting school uniform.

In the summer it was the skirt you had made in needlework, with no thought to how it would look on a curvy figure the picture looked great on the flat mannequin. Box pleats are easy to do, advice on how they will look on you is another matter. Still there are certain things you have to learn in life, the hard way.

Cross Dressing

The feel of women's clothing is a lot nicer than men's. To feel silky pants or thongs on smooth skin, a matching bra, top and skirt is heaven, stockings and garter belt or hold ups complete the look.

To run Your hand over this feast of softness, caressing their flesh with an overload of sumptuousness, rubbing your stockings over theirs, rubbing Your soft leather against their rock hard cocks, as they watch themselves in a mirror.

My maid is a TV. she dresses to make My bed in the mornings, to Hoover the Chamber and tidy the dressing room. Dusting seems beyond her unless she is chivvied along, though she complains about how much dust there is and when the room was recently refurbished, the room edges and under the bed had enough dust to fill the Hoover.

Now you might say that it was My job to get her to do the job properly, well if that was what she wanted, it's not what I expect to do. I don't enjoy maid training. I don't see the point in running around after a maid, picking fault, real or imaginary, just so the maid can be punished. I expect a proper job to be done and a proper session will be given as reward.

Mind I do like My slaves cheeky, she is cute and cheeky...Also very good at practical things like fitting dishwashers and coping with broken showers, her talents outweigh the small inconveniences, there are plenty that can redo the things she misses and if it is possible, she will come running to help when asked, even though she is a very busy business man. she will dress in lovely silky clothes, very slutty with thigh boots, wig and depending on time, make up. I use her in some of My sessions, but she has an aversion to hairy men, which can be a problem sometimes.

The cafe was used by lots of boys and young men, also some students from the local well-known private school. As they had 'money', they thought they were better than us, though some would talk to us giggling girls for a laugh, just as sport. One or two pretty girls got to go out with them, a few more the honour to be taken to the toilets to indulge in some consensual sex. I don't know anyone who had a lasting relationship with one of these boys, but I did have the honour of some fumblings with one of the spotty youths.

The number of boys expelled from that school seemed to be quite high, but I think it was just because the school was high profile. Did I really know one or two of them...?

One day I was alone in the cafe, my mates were not in that day and I got chatting to an older boy, well man really. I had seen him in the cafe a lot and just ogled him from afar. Older men used to like me for some reason. I felt very flattered when he said he had the afternoon off and would I like to go for a drive. As I was bored it only took a bit of cajoling on his part. Talking of nothing much, but him flattering me, put me off the scent of his intentions. When I realised that he just wanted to get his wicked way with my virginal body, I fought like a wildcat. The front seat of a car was not how I wanted to lose my virginity.

The fight was intense, I don't know where I got the strength to pry his fingers from my clothes, but I managed to. He seemed to accept that I wasn't going to lay with him and then we just talked, lulled into a false sense of security, I relaxed a bit. I hadn't banked on him being such a randy git with a passion for virgins, so the next lunge at me was a bit unexpected, but I fought some more and made it out of the car. Walking home with no idea where I was was better than being with him. He sat in the car for a while planning his next strategy. Not that it took him long, for as I learnt at a later date, this was his sport, the way he got his kicks, and he was often in court for rape, though he mostly seemed to get away with it, discrediting the girls name in the process. A lot of girls didn't bother going to the police as you were made out to be a slag in those days.

He pulled up alongside me, crawling along in the car, finding out if I knew the way back and trying to convince me that he would leave me alone, if I got back in the car. He would take me back to the cafe, he eventually convinced me and I think because it was getting late and I had to be home was the deciding factor. So in I hopped, sitting hugging the door as he sped off.

Silly me, he grabbed my clothes as he screeched to a halt and this time I couldn't fight him off.

Poor inadequate male made my first time as unpleasant as he could. In the end I just lay there, thinking, if I don't fight he won't get much enjoyment, that seemed to do the trick and he was soon taking me back to civilization. Dropping me back at the cafe with a thanks and see you again soon.

I don't think so pal.

No I didn't go to the police.

Rape scenes.

Lots of people enjoy these scenes. From the soft playful words of 'I'm going to rape you 'to the full blown brutal fighting off affairs. But both parties are consensual to this. Kidnapping can be part of it, but there are also other reasons someone likes to be kidnapped.

When my exams were due, my father put his foot down, 'no more baby sitting' until I knuckled down and did some revision. My exams were due shortly and though I was in the A stream of the schooling system, I wasn't an intelligent pupil. I found things hard to take on board. The saying is 'in one ear out the other.' Apart from things that really interested me, like housecraft, needlework, English and art...I was such a domesticated soul. I turned my hand at doing the housework at home. Not like now, where I only do it if no one else is around to do it.

TEASE ME, PLEASE ME, WHIP ME, BEAT ME

At a push, if I could have been given the choice, I would have taken a couple of subjects. But I had to take EIGHT GCE's. Life was so unfair, I couldn't even take both needlework and housecraft, life was soo unfair. The kids my father taught could take as few as they wanted. I only wanted to take the ones that would help me in my chosen career.

No I didn't think about being a Dominatrix in those days.

An argument ensued with my father standing firm. It didn't matter that I was being relied upon to look after some children while their parents went to work. My keen sense of honour was at stake here to baby-sit, and I had promised, so nothing was going to stop me. I went upstairs stomping on each one and crying, but plotting what I was going to do.

I formulated a plan, ok he said I couldn't baby sit, if I did he would find out, so I wouldn't baby sit, but neither would I stay at home, grabbing a few things I then crept out of the house, fearful of my Father hearing, then legged it to the house I was to be sitting at. I had been sitting for a few years and they were friends. I explained that I couldn't sit and how sorry I was, that I was going to run away from home, not keep in touch with my family, but would contact them to say if I was ok, if that was alright with them. They tried to talk me out of it, but the headstrong cuss that I am, proved to them this was the only way that I could get what I wanted.

I hitched a ride. I didn't know where I was going; I don't even know how I got there. But I ended up in a small town about twenty miles away.

It was still light as I got there, I found a café, sat and made a coffee last, wondering what I was going to do with myself. Feeling very sorry for myself, and blaming my father for this mess. I wasn't going to back down, lose face, never.

Always the friendly one, I got talking to some boys, they bought me more coffee and then I off loaded my tales of woe onto them, they came up with lots of suggestions and one by one they drifted home, till at last one boy was left. As his parents weren't due home that night, I went to stay at his house. A very nice well brought up boy that had no ulterior motive, bar putting a roof over my head.
We talked most of the night, trying to work out what I was going to do.

I lasted a few weeks, making friends and sleeping wherever I could. I got in touch with my babysitting friends who said my mother would talk to me.... That my father had thought about it and would allow me to leave school if I had a job to go to. So home I went for a week or so, then off to London I went to start a career as a mothers help.

CHAPTER SEVEN

London to a yocal was...different.   I was ensconced in a house looking after the needs of a family. I wasn't ready for that so it didn't work out. After three months I left and went to Hampstead to look after the most enormous baby I had ever seen. She was so fat that at a year old, she would just sit there and do nothing, if she fell over she couldn't get back up again, but would just scream and wave arms and legs like a turtle on its back. Not having enough knowledge to change this child's life, I felt very constricted and didn't last long there either.

I was standing in the underground, tears running down my cheeks, somehow I had managed to leave one job, before I could start at the next...Not wanting to go home and I had a week to go before I started the next.

A guard came up to me all concerned and took me under his wing. I had nothing to lose, and went home with him. Talk about taking my life in my hands.

He was living with his wife and a lodger. His wife didn't think it strange that he had brought a waif home with him. They hadn't got much but shared everything with me, I realise now how much they put themselves out for me.
Their lodger was a member of a local chapter, and we got it together instantly and I was his. We had

a fantastic week together and I went out with him for the rest of my stay in London. Things got very involved between us and he asked me to marry him, but I was too young to marry.

The chapter were a fantastic crowd and I had great fun with them. It was a great learning curve for me and I don't regret a minute of my time with them.

My baby-sitting family need help with their household and I decided to go and work for them, I loved every minute of my time there. He was a property developer and she was a croupier, I knew the kids and loved them, but I was still in My home village, it was a bit defeatist going back home, but still I was seeing My friends and things were familiar. Life was interesting; I was visiting properties with my boss and meeting new people.

For years I had walked around with nothing on my feet, I also did it a lot in London, It wasn't out of place there, and in the village, though I was strange, people were used to it. I often got things in my feet but thought nothing of it.
Once while walking through a house with my employer, balancing on the rafters, there were no floorboards, I stood on a nail, right through my heel. I thought nothing of it, just carried on.... and in London I was always getting glass in my feet but just used to pick the bits out.

TEASE ME, PLEASE ME, WHIP ME, BEAT ME

There were plans being made to emigrate to Spain, I was so excited, I was going with them, sunshine, warmth a new life, I couldn't wait. I bought new suitcases and lots of new stuff. But.... I started to feel off colour, I soldiered on, a bit like my dad in that way, he always went to work, didn't have a day off even when he had the flu, well maybe one day with the flu.

It got to the stage that I couldn't work any longer and got sent to the doctors, I had the kissing disease, wasn't I the lucky one. I went home and my lovely parents looked after me. But time was passing and I couldn't wait to go back to work, so as soon as I felt a little better off I trotted and got into the swing of the move again, but disaster struck and I soon started to feel off colour again. I was slowly going a bright shade of yellow; I couldn't believe it when I was diagnosed with jaundice. So back home to my mums I went.

Our doctor was a funny little man, with a thing about grandfather clocks; every time he came to see us he would spend ten minutes talking about our clock and five with the patient.

I wasn't getting any better, in fact I felt worse and the doctor wasn't noticing that his normally lily white patient was getting persistently more yellow ...the yellow bed sheets might not have helped.
One night when I was curled up and sobbing for England with the pain, the doctor was called. I had a very fast trip to the hospital, where I amazed

my family with my vibrant colour. My fetching yellow eyes dull against the white pillows, clashing with my strawberry blond hair. My freckles lost in the manky yellow tone of my skin. Well there has to be one blessing doesn't there?

The doctors at the hospital couldn't cope with me, the illness was advanced and I needed specialist treatment so I was to be shipped to a bigger hospital. While waiting for the ambulance, I had a visit from the vicar who wanted to give me communion. Now when your liver has been damaged to the extent mine was you don't even need a sniff of alcohol, something the vicar couldn't understand! And he went off more than a little huffy, muttering under his breath.

A little while later I had a slow trip in an ambulance with lights flashing, slow because I couldn't be jolted, I hadn't realised the seriousness off it all till then.
Me clutching a sick bowl and worrying about my mother following behind in her car.

I was isolated, total bed rest and lots of trainee doctors prodding and poking me, that was my life for the next couple of months.

After a period of time, the doctors realised that my bowels had not been open. It's something I just couldn't do without the right conditions, i.e. a loo, bed pans are the spawn of the devil, just peeing in one is an indignity and some things needed to be private. A commode was found for me, and I gave a very small white specimen, but nothing more. So after much discussion, I was allowed to walk ten steps to the loo. I went as quickly as I could before they changed their minds, did the business and got back to bed, where I was confronted by a horrified doctor who was not happy with the nurse who had allowed me to go, contaminating the loo, letting me out of bed and not getting a specimen, but I was smiling at least.

Scat

Some like scat. I don't do it, but can order others to do it.

Liking to see it emerge, to drop onto their body's, have it smeared over them, to smear it over the givers body, face. some like to eat it, warm or cooked. Forced to chew, swallow, savour the smell. For some its an indignity, for others a liking.

Steroids bloated me, and my self-consciousness was pushed aside as the doctors probed me all over. One-day spiders veins were being explained to them. They were told that if you had over a certain amount, this was not good, so one by one they all looked me over and counted, frightening the life out of me as they all came up with well over the amount that was quoted.

Time went on, I got very excited as there was talk of me being moved into the main ward, no more looking at everyone through the glass, no more being in a fish bowl.
The only thing that really changed for me, when I joined the others was that I was able to talk to everyone.

As I got better, I became more conscious of the things that were happening to me, as I was still confined to bed, I had my lost my free will, couldn't even go to the loo without asking. Waiting for a nurse to answer your bell, or if you waited till one came into the ward, you still had to wait as she would more than likely forget...
Eating when given food, woken early, washing when given water. That was one thing that irked me, being given an inch of water to wash in, clean your teeth, just to freshen up with until you can go to the bathroom... Bathroom, did someone mention the bathroom? The place I was not allowed to go, I was still on bed rest.

Begging, pleading, threatening to take myself there did no good, I was still only allowed an inch, once in the morning and once just before visitors arrived, very occasionally a really kind nurse would take pity on me and fill my little bowl a bit more, I was so pathetically grateful

TEASE ME, PLEASE ME, WHIP ME, BEAT ME

Control.

I have to be in control of all around Me. I love people to do things for Me, expect it, as it gives them pleasure, they may do it as they like, but if they do it wrong I tell them the way I want it redone.

I like to be given choices if I am being taken out. I can let people think they are making decisions for Me, but I have the last say. I like people to do the ground work for Me, looking things up, running around, getting things for Me, shopping etc, carrying My bags, opening doors all the courteous things, and lighting My cigarettes.

I live most of My life running slaves, I have a few, I love the adoration and the different types of play I get with them, they are all different but mainly cheeky. I do love a cheeky slave.

I have clients who are in control in their working life, having to think for others, order others about, making decisions and having the weight of responsibility on their shoulders, deadlines to meet and peoples safety in their hands, a lot of pressure from a lot of angles and the pressure is great on them, they need to have the control taken from them, so they can relax. High-powered jobs come with a price, if you can't find a way to relax the pressure can build up and it has to go somewhere or it will explode. Maybe a nervous breakdown.

Playing golf, flying, sport, you need to find what relaxes you, but giving someone else total control of your mind, even if for a little while takes the pressure off. they can then return to a normal, for them, life, free from the stress build up.

Time rolled on and after a liver biopsy that said my liver had a little more life back in it. It had rejuvenated and I was getting a bit pinker. I was allowed to go home, still bed rest though. Here I was allowed as much water as I wanted to wash in, and had my friends visiting me. Though one friend came to visit asking if she could use my new suitcases, to emigrate to Spain with my employers...My God, the cow. My dream in tatters. I understood that I had been ill for four months that things change and they needed to have someone to look after the children, but she was rubbing salt into the wound.

After nine months I went back for another biopsy and my liver had nearly fully recovered. So after a couple more months it was back to work for me.
I went to Sussex this time, looking after a household and a little boy. There I was given the very same opportunity to go to Spain with the family, fate was looking after me.

I had a handsome marine for a boyfriend who was introducing me to the joys of sex. My life was good. The preparations for Spain were moving nicely, I was happy to leave my boyfriend, but my employer was concerned. Every time I went out to meet this chap my room would be trashed, pictures moved, things strewn all over the room, things smashed. My employers, concerned about this, could only surmise that I had a poltergeist. That was not the worry. They wanted to know why I had one. It is common for teenagers in turmoil to produce the electrical energy to open these channels, it didn't really worry me, just puzzled me.

They employed a private detective to follow my boyfriend, I knew nothing of their plans till one day my boss sat me down to talk to me. Explaining what they had done, I started to become indignant, prying into my life, how dare they. They told me that all the time I had been meeting my fella; he had been on compassionate leave, as his wife had just had a baby. Not giving me time to digest this, he asked me what I was going to do. Going to do? What did he mean, I hadn't a clue, so I asked him at the same time as having a go at him for interfering in my life. This had nothing to do with him, and as I was quite happy to leave everything and go to Spain why did he want to know what I was going to do....
A shouting match ensued with me being furious that he had interfered in my life. That he had thought this chap was going to influence my plans to go with them or was he just worried about me. I didn't know, all I knew was that he was telling me to make a choice, did I still want to go to Spain... oh course I did, what a silly question. But the way

he kept asking me, bugged me, he was goading me, he didn't really want a soiled person looking after his family. I snapped, and said I wouldn't go with them, he had got his way. I hadn't even had a chance to digest the news he had given me, and I was out of a job, because he then said if I wasn't going with them, I had better leave the house now. Shit. What was I going to do now?

I moved into a bed and breakfast until I could sort myself out, I made a few friends and started another relationship; I had blown my Marine out and let him get on with his new family.

My new partner was offered work in a new location; guess where... it was back to Somerset for me. Was I ever going to get away from that County? It seemed I was destined to stay there most of my life.

We got ourselves a flat, and started life with nothing, not even a bed and carried on life like that. The bare basics, a bed but no covers, sitting on the floor and cooking with one pan, soup and vegetable stew can get boring.

He was very hot headed, and we rowed a lot, and then his nasty side emerged. He became violent. As I was pregnant by this time I had to stick things out, but running out of the house to get away from someone intent on battering you, when your eight months pregnant, is a bit awkward. I wasn't going to stand there all the time and just let him take pot shots at me. I don't enjoy being given pain.

So when my daughter was six weeks old I did a runner. I found myself work, a live in housekeeping job, they didn't mind my baby being there and things were great until my ex found me, so I had to move on again.

Another housekeeping job, this time looking after a single man and his young son. We settled in well, and as time progressed, we became a family. Still in Somerset. Though we moved about a couple of times. We went on to have a daughter together.
My second daughter never got to see my lovely father, as he died a few weeks before she was born. True to form this wasn't a straightforward time for me. When I learnt my father was very ill, I had been subjected to bed rest, oh God not again, I had high blood pressure, and was strongly advised not to put myself at risk and go and see him. Not one to take direction I set off.

A shell of his former self my lovely father, making an effort to make things easy for me. He made such an effort to give me a good memory to go home with. It must have taxed his reserves.

On reaching home, I was full of foreboding; I rang the hospital and was told to phone my mother... Who told me my father had died.

The day of the funeral arrived, and just as I was leaving home to say my last goodbyes I had another phone call to say I had to leave straight away and book myself into the hospital, as my blood pressure was dangerously high. In tears I explained that I couldn't, and why, and was told to come as soon as possible afterwards.

My new partner was as placid as my previous partner was fiery, but wanting my own way a lot caused a few problems. I worked at various jobs to keep the house together as my partner worked when he felt like it. I was always having to field his phone calls. He was a very good craftsman and in demand and did a fantastic job if you could get him to work.

We were offered jobs at a private girls school, him odd jobs, me helping to cook. I used to love cooking, nowadays I prefer others to cook for Me, or go out to eat, though hunger has meant that I will rustle something up quickly. Oh I will cook for My mother though that may be because I can whiz through the kitchen and rustle up a proper meal at the speed of light, or starve waiting for her to laboriously work her way through the ingredients.

I have people that will cook for Me, be they just house slaves or chefs. I can have friends round and call on My naked chef to prepare and serve the meal, or call on My maids to do the serving and entertain us. Washing up is a dirty word, as is cleaning up, so it's handy to have a few bodies around to do the nasty stuff. maids like to be exhibited in front of people. they like to be looked at, dressed in their uniforms, maid's outfits, heels and wigs. some like to be ridiculed, slapped and taunted, humiliated and used. some are more serious than others. I don't play games with My slaves, they work and get rewarded, I don't run around after them, finding fault and punishing them for their misdemeanours, is pointless in My eyes. I don't talk a lot, don't shout and holler, just expect them to work well. I check up on them every so often, to make sure its being done as I like, giving advise as to the way I want it done, so they are getting My attention.

CHAPTER EIGHT

We moved into a tiny village, in Somerset again, on a high hill that meant when it snowed the girls didn't have to go to school, as the mini bus that took them there couldn't skid down the pretty tree lined, toboggan slope of a narrow road. Mind we could have walked up to the main road, but if we did that the bus might not be there and who wants a wasted journey, (tongue in cheek). It was more fun building snowmen.

After a few more years, I got itchy feet, my life was boring, I was fed up, depressed and not doing an awful lot apart from working and reading a lot. Anything sci-fi or soppy books, Mills and Boon were a favourite, I began to want a romantic partner, I wanted a life as in the books. I was moody, not happy and I began to take it out on the kids, I had to change my life, get away and start afresh.
I moved to Bournemouth, wow not Somerset.
I loaded my car and set off for a flat I had not seen, but had been promised. An adventure for the unhappy girls, their toys and personal bits loaded high in my car.

We got lost, I always get lost but that adds to the thrill of things. I have a sat nav now but don't always believe it, I keep challenging it, its not always right, mind it might help if I learnt how to program it properly, but why do I need to learn, I usually have slaves around to do it.

TEASE ME, PLEASE ME, WHIP ME, BEAT ME

When we arrived at the flat, tired, I was told that my flat had been given to someone else. Oh boy, here we go homeless yet again, but this time I had children with me. The landlady said in her broken English, that she did have another flat though, lucky me... bigger and more money, she had me by the short and curlies. OK, if I wanted beds for my babies I had to take it.
She was a typical landlord, not doing repairs and taking your deposit when you leave even though I redecorated before I left.

I had a great time there. I made friends with the lady who took my flat, she had two girls close to my girls' age, and we all got on great. We went through a lot and ended up sharing another flat six months down the line when our winter let lease was up and we had to move out.

I got a cleaning job and got on great with the old ladies, running around doing their chores, I had a favorite, a little old lady. She was about four foot ten, stooped and tiny and had such an innocent cheeky face and manner, but you had to be careful when you walked into her room as she would shed little rabbit droppings from her knickers wherever she walked, being partially sighted she was never aware of this, though they must have squished under foot, and her being deaf, telling her loudly would have embarrassed her, so it was easier just to brush them up every day.

I progressed to doing the cooking and laundry. Back to the home making drudge, but it was something I still enjoyed.

I got myself a CB radio, it was in the days when it was illegal and I was getting a buzz from that fact and also making lots of new friends.

One day a new, very sexy voice came over the airwaves, I spent a few hours trying to arrange a meet with the voice, he took some persuading, but gave in eventually, I sat and waited and waited, and waited, a few hours later, he said he was in my road, so I went to the door to help him find the flat. It was freezing and there was snow on the ground and as he walked to the door he slipped over, I picked him up in more than one way that day, he never left, my toy boy. Someone who was to cause me so much pleasure and aggravation for the next nine years.

We all moved into the new flat when the lease was up on the old one, my friend, her children, my partner and my children, a bit cramped, but a happy time. I was working to support us; I was still supporting my man, why does nothing change. I became pregnant, and on my way to my very last shift at work, on my trial bike, I hit some oil on a bend and decided to wear the road as an extra layer of clothing. It scared the shit out of some onlookers. Well, seeing a heavily pregnant woman sliding towards them with a bike on top of her has that effect. Picked up, patted down and assuring everyone that I was okay, I set off again to work, I couldn't let the ladies down I had to cook their supper. The adrenalin had kicked in and I just brushed off the fact my arse was red raw and hanging out of my trousers. I got an old dear to pick off the biggest bits of gravel, then freshened up and carried on with feeding the hungry hoard. Mind I took to my bed when I got home, and my eldest daughter cleaned me up. By this time I just let go and the adrenalin had calmed down and I was a quivering wreck, scared that I had harmed my unborn child.

My youngest is mad, unruly, wayward and lovable, the fall must have caused that.... Well I have to blame something. In the last couple of weeks at home, life was a bit boring, but one day a man came to liven it up for me.

I was having a rest one afternoon, when my daughter went into the kitchen to see a man there. She asked him who he was and what he wanted. He said he had come to empty the meter, we had a fifty pence electric meter. She came running to me. Thinking it strange as it had only been emptied a couple of weeks before; I entered the kitchen to find him putting our money into his pocket. How dare he, I shouted at him, and he turned tail and ran. With me in hot pursuit. I chased him down the flights of stairs yelling and swearing at him, I grabbed him and was going to kick him down the stairs but did a back track when he turned around to face me and threaten me. I watched him run down the street with a cyclist in hot pursuit, and was told he jumped into a taxi to avoid the cyclist catching him.

All I can hope is that it took all My fifty pence's to pay the cab fare. But I'm sure there were some left over to pay for his next fix.

My daughter was born, and my partner, always helpful, was always taking on jobs that it was possible for me to do, when he couldn't be fussed to do them. One being a video film hire delivery, on the motorbike. He loved this job, he would send me out to deliver and pick up the films while his mates and him sat and watched them, he had a lot of mates and they all needed refreshments when I got back from my round, they loved the fact I would run round waiting on them, their own little slave.

The school holidays arrived and I took the children out to a theme park as a treat. We had a nice time and some excitement on the way back; as a lot of fire engines were racing in the direction we were going. We laughed and joked and said they were heading for our place. There was a road block so we couldn't go the way we wanted, so we went by a back road, but when we couldn't go any further, we got out to look, a passer by told us our block of flats was on fire. With trepidation I ran round the corner to see flames escaping from my windows and firemen up a ladder aiming water into the rooms. Our friend who owned the sweet shop opposite us took care of the girls while I pieced together the facts, that someone had broken into the house, stolen the video and anything else of worth and legged it across the roof tops, but not before raking out the embers of a fire I had going in the living room.

We lost everything, photos, family heirlooms, clothes...Everything. My partner's family were fantastic to us during this time, and his brother heard about the fire on the news and left work to be with us before the firemen had left.

My daughter was less than a year old, and we were homeless again...Well not quite, we did have a camper van, the whole family rallied around with clothes and personal items, a place to sleep, friends helped clothe and look after the children, the local church helped with some money, everyone was fantastic. We went into a bed and breakfast until we could get another place.

Lumpy beds, out by nine back at six, no cot for the baby and unfriendly owners. Our camper came into its own then, it was our best buy, it kept us from walking the streets and gave us a decent nights sleep occasionally. My older girls went to stay with my previous partner, and came back when we had a new place to live.

I became very depressed at this time, it was a downward slope. I had a nice house and great kids but I couldn't enjoy life. My partner had his own life, earnt his own money and spent it on any new hobby he took up; he had a harem of women that I chose to ignore because I loved him. I was still going out to work, but not allowed any freedom, he was very jealous and didn't like me getting attention, what was good for the goose wasn't good for the gander.

My girls were growing up, my oldest starting to become a woman. My partner started to take an interest in her. I didn't want to think that he was acting in an unbecoming manner around her, my depression blocking these things out. It was only when I was called to her school that it came out that he had been touching her and was suggestive to her. I was in a quandary, I wanted to believe her but I loved my partner, surely he wouldn't molest her, torn two ways, I was willing to talk things through with him and others and was persuaded to give him the benefit of the doubt, to the detriment of my relationship with my daughter.

We carried on with the rocky relationship nothing really changing, but my daughter becoming more unhappy and moody. I should have been stronger and split from him, as I had always found it easy enough in the past to up sticks and move on, but I think my lethargy had taken a deep hold and was getting worse with each new set back. The doctor couldn't or wouldn't help and I was just going through the motions of life.

My poor children had a hard time in lots of ways, money was tight and I was making them cycle miles to school, their mother was working many hours to hold things together and she was no help to them, couldn't really hold a conversation with them or muster up the energy to make life fun for them.

A move was in order; a change might help, so we moved closer to the coast. Nothing changed, we had just moved and I had an operation which meant I had to stay off my leg for six weeks so my partner found me a sitting down job in a taxi office, how thoughtful of him...

His latest fad was shooting, which was fun, I seemed to take to it, even the girls liked it, though I wasn't allowed to practice much. He decided that we could sell refreshments from the camper van, so my time was spent in there, apart from when I had a competition, I managed to get a few medals for shooting and all his practice made him quite good to.

As it was cheaper to make your own ammunition, casting the lead bullets, redoing primers, loading powder, and crimping became my job, well all the practice stuff anyway, his competition ammo was done by him.

Things weren't getting any better with my depression, and being used as a workhorse meant that the kids were suffering. The allegations came up again against my partner and this time with my middle daughter. The oldest had left home and married. After a talk with her we went to the police who brought charges against him.

During this time he made life for us as uncomfortable as he could, from taking money from us, threatening us and putting our lives at risk. I was a gibbering wreck though people didn't know how bad I was as I have always put on a good front and taken others troubles as worse than my own and helped them. The week of the court case came, and the girls were subjected to humiliation, my eldest had her sexual history dragged out. The girls were ridiculed his barrister knew his job. We were all dragged through the coals, my ex's long time girlfriend sat next to me in court and giggled and talked throughout, making us look bad, a calculated action, he lied about all the things he had done and provided false alibis for the things he was being accused of doing to me...he got off, then had the gal to say we were only doing this to claim the money we could have claimed for attending. We didn't ...he did.

My time with him was over, no more verbal humiliation, being used as a meal ticket, a slave and an occasional punch bag.

A friend helped pay for a few of us to go to Spain on holiday. Well he did at the time, we had to pay afterwards when we got served with papers, threatening to take us to court, he had paid nothing, we ended up paying for him as well as our own.

TEASE ME, PLEASE ME, WHIP ME, BEAT ME

There My youngest decided to change her name totally, missing out her first and last name. She didn't know what he had done, but knew what he was causing to the household he didn't care that the children, his child was being hurt.

We had a great time, on a budget though. The sun and swimming was a good therapy for us. We all managed to relax. We were in awe of the fishes that swarmed around us when we swam and the beautiful countryside. The kids became as brown as berries and the local food agreed with us, though the tight budget meant that the cheap cigarettes were worked into the budget. The kids wouldn't have wanted two grumpy females tearing their hair out.

The flight home was a little apprehensive, as it was back to a life that we weren't sure about. Were we going to get more hassle? We arrived late at night, the kids were tired, but we knew we could sleep on the long journey home. We stood by the conveyor waiting for our bags to come through, we waited and waited, waited some more, then when everyone had gone our bags came out. Off we trotted through the green lane, nothing to declare, and were pounced on by a customs man who asked us to follow him, why? Lack of money had meant we didn't bring anything back with us. The youngest child was dead on her feet, all of us tired, but we had to make the most of what was happening to us. We were asked the usual questions and our bags searched. My bag of prescription drugs inspected and our male friend taken away for questioning. There was nothing to find and after a time we were let go.

Piecing things together afterwards we came to the conclusion that this was my ex partners work, his parting shot at causing us as much inconvenience as he could. Though how he could put two young children through that I don't know, but that was his sense of humour.

As he left me in debt and my health was beginning to suffer I had to find work I could do. I have a problem with my knees and nursing was taking its toll on them. The many hours I was putting in at work meant my oldest was looking after the younger children, and no one was very happy.

I moved house to get away from the memories. Not very far away, but I soon made new friends in the street.

I felt I was in dire straights and needed to do something to get some money together, limited as to what I could do, I looked into joining an escort agency. My new friends could help if I had a job by taking the children out of the way, giving them a treat, one I could never have afforded before, they were none the wiser, so I saw a few clients and paid my debts off. I didn't need to work for long as I was purely in it to pay my debts off. I didn't waste the money, though the children did get treats that they wouldn't have got before.

TEASE ME, PLEASE ME, WHIP ME, BEAT ME

My health was getting worse. My mobility was impaired and I needed some one with me all the time. I couldn't walk far and would gently topple to one side if I hadn't got some one to steady me. I was in constant pain, and became addicted to the painkillers I was throwing down my neck, so I weaned myself off them and managed the pain and used weaker painkillers.

CHAPTER NINE

I met my husband at this time. He was ruled by his alcoholic drug-taking son, at his beck and call for money or anything that he wanted done. He was insanely jealous of me, and not too many years younger than me.

Our marriage was a sham as I felt I was forced into it. I never wanted to get married, I was happy living with him, but he was adamant that that was what he wanted. I was looked after physically but accused by his son of taking all his money, which irked me, as I had my own money and paid the bigger share of the bills...yet again....

One day he came to me in tears, very upset, and said that his son had bullied him into agreeing to divorce me, he always did as his son wanted. It was no skin off my nose, so I agreed. Nothing changed in the relationship between us, which really annoyed his son.

We still did things together, though he had moved out. That suited me, as I like my own company better than being around people all the time. We went on holidays with my daughter. It was on a holiday that I noticed that he wasn't himself, nothing I could put a finger on, but his aura was different, I sensed he was ill.

TEASE ME, PLEASE ME, WHIP ME, BEAT ME

I was seeing a consultant who could do nothing for me apart from drain the floating bits of bone that were grating in my knee caps. Arthritis. That eased the pain for a while. He referred me to a new consultant who gave me the choice of a new procedure. Drastic as it was I took it. It meant that my leg needed to be broken and the tendons cut. With trepidation I had the operation. I was buzzing when I came round from it; I had far less pain than before. I came home to be looked after by my daughter who had left home and a useless younger daughter who had not grown up enough to think of anyone but herself.

I was confined to bed for a while as my muscles had wasted through the years of not being able to walk yet alone exercise much, getting to the loo was difficult, turning over in bed ditto but things got better as the days went on, until the day it became apparent my ex husband couldn't cope at home anymore.

I had taken him to have a few tests months before and we had been given the news that he had cancer. When he knew this, he carried on till the last, living life normally, but not really accepting that he was going to die, not even telling his family. As he wanted to die at home with me and the time was getting close, he moved back in. I was more mobile and my daughter was a great help, we both looked after him, every day he was getting worse. It was time to tell his family. His daughter and children came to visit, a very harrowing time, but no sign of his son.

We treated him as we normally would, making jokes of his infirmities, picking him up when he fell, telling him to take more water with his whiskey wheeling him in his chair to visit friends. He accepted near the end that he was going to die. my cast had come off and I was able to do more for him, but one night his breathing got so bad I panicked and not being able to get in touch with his nurse I called an ambulance and his daughter. His lungs were full, there was nothing they could do he didn't get his wish of dying at home, but I was by his side all the time, which was his wish.

CHAPTER TEN

It was about this time that My friend introduced Me to the world of BDSM.

Using the resources from inside Me I decided that was how I was going to make My living.

I went to a local sex shop and spent far too much money but not enough really.
I wasn't versed with the fact that you can raid your kitchen for a lot of tools, we all adapt or use kitchen utensils, and a trip round a local D.I.Y. store is pervy heaven. So much to choose from, not really knowing what I was going to do or how I was going to do it, I advertised in the local paper. It had to be under escorts and the wording had to be vague, so I was pounced on by all the usual suspects that have to see new advertisers. The chaps that never go to see the same escort twice, sometimes I saw them. I did get some clients for Domination though.

I fumbled My way through the sessions putting on a front and hoping I was doing the right thing...so nervous that I'm sure My inexperience showed and it put people off coming to see Me. But a few could see My potential liked the way I worked and are still with Me today.

If I was on the outside, looking in on the newly starting Me, I would have been terrified for the clients and probably cringing at how badly I was doing the job. I know that when I'm observing newcomers to the scene playing at venues, I feel horror, but there is nothing I can do. They are used to playing together that is the way they play and if you interfere you are saying you know more than they do. Which might be so in some scenes. Though not everyone wants to learn things, as they know everything they need to... Myself I'm like a sponge, I want to learn and learn more, I'm still reading and asking questions and watching others.

Absolutely petrified every time the phone rang. Then not understanding some of the phrases that were being used, but things were simple once they were explained to me. I read avidly, absorbing all I could. I found that this was something that actually stayed in My brain.... I can't work the DVD controls or anything electrical, but I can use My hands and mouth, and any other part of Me to bring exquisite pleasure to My paying clients.

I joined some BDSM sites and got inundated with offers from slaves. Now I had no idea how to use a slave, I had always done the running around and though I had lots of jobs for them to do, it didn't seem right, not doing them myself. How did I treat a slave?

I decided on a very pretty boy who had blond hair flopping over his eyes, tall and fit. Willing to do anything, so the kitchen started to be done. his lungs were clogged with dust as he sandpapered the kitchen units. I dressed in My leather for him, sat and talked or stayed close by on the computer. I listened to him talking about his problems. He gave Me some hints, I learnt from him. He told Me about Munches. The meeting of like-minded people. Where people meet and exchange ideas or just talk about normal life. They were fun, people brought in rope and tied others up, they brought in anything that took their fancy and did demonstrations. I was learning and able to put these things into practice with My guinea pigs, oops sorry, clients.

I went to My first Munch with My daughter, slave had told Me it wasn't a dress up event but daft Me went in a Basque, daughter was dressed in vanilla style. Looking through the door I saw I was decidedly overdressed, I had a coat on, and hid under it. Daughter took pity on Me and suggested we change clothes, lucky Me. The Basque fits our size and her clothes fitted Me. More at ease after a change in the toilet, I got talking to a few and as the ice broke I began to relax. Slave wasn't there, he has only been once and works shifts so it's difficult or so he says, I say he could come if he wanted.

At a future meeting I got talking to a very unhappy boy, he was so sweet, he was talking about fisting, something that grabbed My interest, I wanted to know all I could about it. I had done a little anal play and found it a big turn on.

I learnt that he was just out of a long-term relationship with his 24/7 Mistress. I couldn't believe the things she had done to him. he was a pain slut and told Me she could drop him as she lashed out without warning. he seemed to like it though. She had total control of his life. She would dictate to his boss that he had to come home when she said. The time didn't matter. Now that was control and he was missing it badly, he couldn't function without it. I couldn't give him that control; all I could give him was the means to have his self esteem built up. It took a while. he was very cheeky, which I love in slaves now, he set the precedence for that.

he taught Me a lot, but things did not go well between us, because he was young, and I'm fifty-three now, he lived about half an hour away and I did not want to intrude in his life, when I knew he had had a busy stressful day at work.
I was too considerate of his wellbeing and health, I was still in nurturing mode, not realising that You can call on slaves at any time. I felt I could not use him willy nilly as he had a life. he was not used for jobs and I just played with him, learning that safety was a very important aspect in BDSM, though some of the things I learnt I found to be over the top, but it was an important lesson to learn as its best to be ultra safe to begin with and then adapt to Your way of working.

he spoke to Me of a meeting place in Bristol, early on in Oour acquaintance, a place that had a fetish market and a playtime in the evening. That sounded good, he drove Me there. I found lots of toys and tools to buy there and as Wwe went every month I soon had spent a lot of money stocking up on tools of the trade. Though through him I learnt that everywhere you go, you can adapt household implements to use for whatever your fetish. I now look at everything with the thought of using it in play, I still buy from the market every month, I never have enough tools, just as every time I go out shopping you can guarantee that I will come back with something pervy.

I was excited about going to the fair, but did not know what to expect, so put on My very confidant head and strutted around the market as if I owned the place, head held high and letting all know that I was a Dominant by My obnoxious manner. It makes Me laugh when I see others doing exactly that now and cringe to think that I was doing that a few years ago.

I made friends and realised that we are all the same, though some are more obnoxious than others. We had a common interest and I could learn from almost every one.

A client came to see Me wanting a hard caning, to bleeding, he had been refused by other Dommes or they couldn't do it. I said I would and he came along. I gave him a good beating, but he wanted more. I could and did do it. I didn't like him much, he was too grovelling and there was something not quite right about him, but I have found that to be the case with some slaves and it makes Me uneasy. I can cope if clients are that way, but not My slaves. So he started to do jobs for Me, more sanding; he would be coughing up the doorframe dust.

I didn't really hit it off with My pretty boy either; there was something that didn't sit right. I didn't know then that You can pick one or more that suits You. he stayed with Me for about a year, then I wouldn't see him any more, I couldn't give him what he really wanted, I didn't know how to play with him the way he wanted, I felt that everything I was doing with him was being taken with complacency, the right vibes were not there. he still to this day keeps asking to come back and I sometimes give him a session, but things have not improved in the fact I can't get any satisfaction from playing with him. I also at that time wouldn't return My other slaves calls. I was not versed in the fact that I can just tell slaves what I want or don't want. I was too caring about their feelings and that I might hurt them, so I just tried to wrangle out of things. he eventually got the hint and I didn't hear from him again. Nowadays I am more confident and only take on slaves that suit Me. I still get many offering their services.

At the moment I have a slave who has been with Me for a couple of years. he valets My car, cleans My oven, paints the fence, cuts the hedge, anything I tell him to do, he came to Me never having anything and not knowing what he wanted. I have brought him on slowly, he can't be marked for obvious reasons, but the urge has taken such a strong hold on him that he now gets very brave and asks to be beaten, knowing that he will go home with some marks to hide, sometimes I deliberately gave him some marks for being so cheeky. he is always asking questions, can never learn enough. Its not a servile relationship he does the jobs I set him and gets a session for doing them, he is not really submissive, just likes the things I do to him.

he likes CBT, Cock and Ball Torture, something I really enjoy doing. It has taken years of experimenting with him to get into the mind space that Wwe are now in. he is able to take more and more each time I see him and now he can take a good paddling, ending with a caning, that leaves some marks that he has to hide from his wife, he likes the excitement of this, though I'm not sure how he does it. he has a nervous laugh that I can bring on with just a look, and I do that quite often, just to un-nerve him. he will clean My car if I am going somewhere special, cut the hedge, paint the fence and break My oven whilst cleaning it. Denying all knowledge and being severely punished for the fact. All with a cheeky grin.

Early on in Oour relationship, I went out with him for a drink, we sat and talked of BDSM. On the way home I got a phone call from him, he was soo cheeky that I turned the car around and met him in a lay-by. Ordering him out of his car I told him to bend over the bonnet of My car, I pulled his trousers down and proceeded to spank his bottom. he was so excited by this fact that he came all over the bonnet of My defenceless Ophelia, as a car was going by. Not best pleased with that he was told to readjust his clothing and find a tissue to clean My baby up, then told he was to come the next day to clean all the evidence away.

I seem to favour spanking by the roadside. One night when My cute young slave and I were coming back from a Munch, I decided he had been extra cheeky and deserving of a spanking, so told him to stop the car in a lay-by. I ordered him out and told him to take his trousers down and lean against the side of the car. he did so, he was in view of passing cars, and I proceeded to make his bottom red. The added thrill of the fact was that it was quite close to where his mother lived. After a few cars had gone by and he was in a nice haze of fluffiness, I allowed him to pull his trousers up and continue to drive Me home.

TEASE ME, PLEASE ME, WHIP ME, BEAT ME

CHAPTER ELEVEN

Rubber

I have a fair amount of rubber, latex. Not the pretty stuff to go to parties in but stuff for My clients to wear, giving them a few layers to put on. Every time I go to the factory I spend a fortune, can't resist it. Shirts, trousers, pants, hoods, skirts and tops, bloomers, chastity devices, a strait jacket, body suits with and without hood, loose and tight, with and without arm restraints, body bags and rubber sheeting, wank bags, stockings, gloves and blindfolds to mention a few; I have two chests full of the stuff. I have a cape skirt, custom made stockings and corset. It gets hot in these clothes and that's the idea of multiple layers.

I have a naughty boy who comes to see Nanny. he is wearing his rubber pants and as he walks through the door he has to drop his trousers and I beat his bottom with a rubber tawse then send him upstairs and dress him in dungarees or encase him in a suit with access holes through which I will abuse any accessible part. he has been a naughty boy and tells Me the things he has done and thought of. I will be wearing My layers of latex and stockings, and will be taunting him with glimpses of My bloomers that reach My knees, and using key words. Describing first My rubber macintosh sliding over My rubber skirt that is hiding Nanny's rubber bloomers. Nanny bending over the tight rubber outlining Nanny's bottom.

The wank bag has to come into action as I lean over My boy and run the cape over his face, using the key words, till he cums.

A party that I attend has some very pretty girls wearing very pretty expensive rubber wear, I would love to wear something like that, but with a figure like Mine its best kept under wraps, so as not to frighten babies and the elderly. I can dream though and one day I have been promised by a friend that she will design a dress for Me that I will get made up by the local manufactures.

I have a chap that likes to experience breath control while wearing rubber. While totally enclosed, and wearing high, high heels, he likes to have a noose put round his neck, then be given poppers till he was so light headed that he would totter on his heels, then be given more, suspended by his neck as he loses balance, hanging by the neck till I let the rope loosen, he is sat down and he can recover, then I do it again. I have to be very careful and watch his body language and breathing all the time. he likes re-breathing and anything to do with breath control.

Plastic

My puppy likes plastic. he wears plastic pants, jogging bottoms and top. The feel of the plastic against his skin is a big turn on for him. I get him to do menial jobs, clean the wet room, the toilets.

TEASE ME, PLEASE ME, WHIP ME, BEAT ME

It is a release for him from the stresses of his life. he also likes breath control.

he brings a plastic bag, which I put over his head as he is chained to the wall, he can breath through the bottom of the bag, but as I have control of this I soon restrict the flow. Twisting the bottom of the bag up till no more air is going in, he is gasping on the little that is in the bag. I let go before he is in too much distress, but build up till he is fighting for breath. Sometimes I will secure the bag around his neck and make a hole to the side of his mouth through which I control the airflow. All the time I am controlling his breathing I and pressing myself against him and stroking him, watching him constantly.

I have a bubble hood, well two really a rubber one and a plastic one. I use the plastic one on him. It's a pretty blue colour. I ordered it with a load of other plastic gear for him. I intend to take him to parties with Me, and as he can't wear his see through gear I bought some plastic jeans and a biker jacket, plus schoolgirl gear and body bags and other gear.

The hoods have two layers, one that is forced to lay flat on the contours of his face as the outer layer is inflated into a bubble, there is a pipe, which goes into his mouth and is attached to a bag that I can use to control his intake. he is either lying or kneeling for this as I can't see his face, can only go on body language, and if the worst happened and he passed out I would have no need to cut him down or undo him from the hindrances of cuffs and chains. Between My knees I can grip him tight, maintain body contact and keep him under control. I have great big black plastic bags, which I put him into. The first time I did it, I put him in it on the floor between My legs, with his head at the mouth of the bag, Me scrunching it up tight. I left him in it, in the pitch black for a while, then started to cover his mouth and nose, stopping his breathing. It got to the stage that he was fighting for air and stretched out in the bag. As he was curled into a ball when I put him in the bag he managed to force his foot through the bottom of this heavy duty plastic. Naughty boy. The next time I used it on him, I put his head the other way up, near the broken part, which I then put My hand through and held his mouth and nose with skin-to-skin contact, and as he stretched, his feet felt no resistance.

I can sit on his face whilst he is in the bag. Easing My posterior into position, Me smiling as he starts to wriggle and squirm, then lifting off allowing him to breath, then clamping My bottom onto his face once again, putting full weight on him, pushing his face deep into the bed, feeling the heat as his breath heats the plastic between My thighs

. Relinquish controlling

I include anal play in tie and tease. A lot of clients come to see me, never having come to see a Dominatrix before; it's a good introduction. When I get a phone call it could be from a client that just wanted sex. I explain I don't do that, but the closest I get to it is tie and tease; a lot don't understand the concept of receiving sensations and not being able to touch. I can understand that to a certain extent as I like to give pleasure, but you have to try most things at least once, to know if you will enjoy it.
A lot won't relinquish control, can't relax enough to enjoy the sensations, they want to touch You sexually, give You pleasure, but they are not there for that reason, unless that is what I want them to do.

While they are there, they can see My chamber and all the things in it, and sometimes they see something that interests them, something they had never really thought about before, or only dreamed about. I can then bring that thought to life.

On one of the sites I advertise on, all the men, well not all as a lot do come to see Me, and some of the women, think that Domination is about pain. Shouting women carrying whips and walking all over men. A few have been enticed to the dark side and some of them have come back to try it a second and third time. they would never admit to others that they have been to see Me, where the working girls get reports on them, I don't...though a few have admitted to meeting Me, not in the line of business though, only one has admitted that. So though many can say what I am like to talk to, I am still the Domme that will beat you up.

Control is a strange thing, if you don't want to relinquish there is no point in coming to see Me. A submissive needs to have the control taken from him he needs another to tell him to do things, let him be mindless and let You have the upper hand. A submissive can have a very demanding job, issuing orders and living the high life, or just be a very gentle person who won't rock any boats. My puppy is a very gentle person, I don't know if he has been all his life, but he can't assert himself in his marriage, and his wife wants a stronger personality for a partner. But in saying that she is quite happy for him to do all the chores, though she won't order him to do them, she is disgusted that he wants to be ordered around and can't understand that he would put up with all the crap she could throw at him quite happily, but when he explained a little of this to her she ran around telling all her friends, who then called him a pervert, well he is, as I am, but not in the way she meant, he works long hours to keep her in a very nice lifestyle, but I think she may have burnt her bridges, as she has made life so intolerable for him, that she may soon have to cut her cloth according to her new income.

he has an assistant who has to arrange his appointments, take any flack from his clients if he has to rearrange, and during a conversation he had with her one day, he was apologising for any crap she would get, she said don't worry that's my job, but he couldn't leave it at that and kept saying sorry, she got so fed up with him in the end that she just put the phone down on him.

My clients are all too happy to do My bidding. If I want to dress them, paddle them, get them on their knees licking My shoes, or making their knees shake with the intensity of being chained while I abuse their bodies in a variety of ways. I have total control of their minds and bodies.
If someone has a fetish then I can control them using this fetish. If its rubber that gives them the good feelings then from the moment they smell the rubber or see it they are Mine, to do, as I want with. When the need has been satisfied they can go back to run their lives happier people.

CHAPTER TWELVE

FOOT FETISH

I love My feet massaged, I love My feet stroked, I love My toes sucked. To rub My stocking-ed feet over someone's face, body cock. To cover a face with both feet, to squeeze their nose between the arches of My feet, scrunching My toes over their eyes, pushing My toes up their noses and into their mouths, first the big toe then each toe after. Feeling their tongues lick around My toes and deep down into the depths, sliding between the toes. Then, them gently sucking as I push all the toes into their mouth, forcing as much of My foot as I can into their mouths.

With shoes on, rubbing the soles along a cock, over balls, squashing them flat against their bodies. Using the toe to push between the balls and separating the balls then pressing hard so the skin is then pushed against the cock base, balls either side of the shoe. Then using the heel to do the same, but digging into the base of the cock stump. The flat sole of My shoe squashing the rock hard cock into his belly. Then, trailing My toe down the cock over the balls along the perineum and teasing the anus. Sliding over the sensitive bud, up between the arse cheeks, then back to the ass hole. Teasing by putting a little pressure then pushing harder, till the tip of My shoe enters and I start to fuck them.

TEASE ME, PLEASE ME, WHIP ME, BEAT ME

I had a chap come to see Me the other day, and he had never fulfilled his fantasies. One of which was Me in Wellington boots. I had never done that before and as I'm not really an outdoors person, well apart from strapping slaves to trees in the forest, I don't possess rubber boots. So he brought a pair of size tens for Me to put My size sevens into, along with some jodhpurs that I eased My ample frame into. I had to taunt him, that I was going to ride My horse up to his range rover, jump off the horse and steal his car, wearing My boots, flaunting them at him all the time, then pull over and rub My boots all over his face. he was dressed in netball gear, and had just left a match in which he was one of the girls, every one had been taunting him, Me included, and when he left he was wearing the things I had been wearing along with his netball gear, hidden by a big jacket.

Spitting

I have come across people that like to be spat at. Hawking in their faces, gathering a big ball of spit and aiming it wherever, mostly into their mouths. Telling them to open their mouths and projecting a stream of spittle into their mouths and telling them to swallow. Aiming it onto their face and watching it slide down, dribbling slowly into their mouths, their eyes transfixed on the bubbles escaping My mouth, watching as it slowly drips down, getting ever closer to their mouths, then feeling the spit sliding over their tongue reaching the back of their throat, not letting them swallow till I say. The degrading feeling they get as I laugh at the sight. Making them feel two inches tall and worthless.

My garden was becoming a mess. Work was becoming hectic. Work on the computer, web cam, phone chats and clients visiting, also I was doing outcalls. One of these outcalls was to a client who needed CP; he was a naughty schoolgirl who had to report to the Headmistress. I chastised him and he was hooked, he needed to keep seeing me. he came to see Me a few times and we got talking. he needed to do something other than his work and as the garden needed a tender touch, he started to nurture it. he put a lot of hours into this, but he has one failing, well more than one really but this one is that he's clumsy, very clumsy. Always hurting himself or breaking some thing, every time he came he would cut his finger, bang his head, drop something on his toe, fall over, it was never ending.

he was laid off from work, a job he loved but was emotionally draining for him, and became very depressed. Every time he came, most days, he would talk to Me, he couldn't get his head around the fact that his health was never going to get better, he did the rounds of hospital visits, with his new and existing illnesses, and he dropped deeper and deeper into depression. he should have known how to cope with it, as that had been his work before. Coming to Me each day was helping him keep his head from going into the depths, his cheeky side coming out. Hiding behind a tree and having a crafty fag, keeping an eye out for Me striding down the garden cane in hand, ready to motivate his ass with a tap or three.

The lawn was looking good, and he was making inroads into the veggie patch, I was giving him free reign the first year he started, as he said he had had an allotment in the past and used to keep his family in veggies all year round, he was not doing things the way I wanted, but if they were to come out satisfactory, then I would allow this...they didn't, he had strange ideas, like putting fresh manure on plants...ouch burnt roots, dead plants...The glut of veggies didn't materialize, every instruction seemed to go in one ear and out the other. Well I did give him the benefit of the doubt that first year.

I did force him to get a hearing aid, which didn't help with the instructions as he always had it out of his ear and was fiddling with it.

Every year he did the veg plot I thought it might get better, but he never really got to grips with it, manure was his thing, he loved to dig it in, spread it over the plants, dilute the deer droppings he had gone into the forest to collect at the dead of night. Was that a black magic ritual? No not really he likes to observe the wildlife and nocturnal activities...he made sure I got the tree pruners in and arranged for My pond to be relined. Now that was a disaster.

A chap, a graduate from a local fishery collage came, he was told what I wanted and he said he could do it. I didn't stand over him and offer advice, I was very good, but he was not doing the job on consecutive days. So My fifty odd fish that had been put in a small holding tank, on hot summer days, with no oxygenating weed or running water started to die. I phoned him and he wasn't concerned, so I put the pump in, and that stopped the loss of life.

He had taken the existing purbeck paving from the edge of the pond and put it in a pile, along with the pile of plants and weed, thus letting the wildlife go somewhere safe till the pond was refilled.

After a few days, he came back and carted off all the rubbish and started on the relining, filling the pond and pissing off for a couple more days. The fish were suffering so I had to put them in the pond, with no further loss of life, but with one strand of weed, floating in a vast space, things looked bleak. The chap came back and put two plants back in the pond, which escaped within two days and were floating on the top. He had started to do the crazy paving around the pond. It broke My heart to see the finished article. He had taken all the little stones to the tip, the work consisted of as much concrete as stone work, the rounded inner edge was uneven, no smooth edge all jutting out rocks, the weathered tops I had told him I wanted kept on top had been put underneath and hidden. I blew My top and told him off, I told him I would never recommend him to anyone, and wouldn't trust him to redo it. I had to get My original chap in to redo the work, which was difficult as the materials weren't there any more. The pond needed a lot of care afterwards to get it back into shape, and new garden slave managed to get it back to its former glory, because by this time old garden slave was languishing in his dark depths.

Beating old garden slave sometimes helped, chivvying him, cajoling him, getting on at him, chastising him, all sometimes helped, but the days he came became fewer and fewer. Threatening him with getting someone else in to do his work didn't rouse him sufficiently, and the day came, after him being with Me for a few years that I had to get someone else in. The garden had suffered enough. So another ex client took his place.

I had become close to him and went to his family get togethers, his family accepted Me and My work...We are all perves in one-way or another. Things became so bad that he secluded himself in his flat, with nothing ever going right for him. Losing his car and driving licence seemed to be the last straw for him, he had always gone out and about in the forest, packing some sandwiches and his camera, off to take pictures of the deer in the forest or night fishing where he always managed to fall in the water.
The garden and work taken from him, what was he to do, sit at home and watch the television,

that's what. his place getting more and more untidy, and him sleeping a lot. his texts and phone calls to Me becoming less frequent. I went to visit him a couple of times, which cheered him a little but he didn't want to go to meetings, munches or Bristol Swamp, there was no helping him. It got to the stage where I said to hell with it, let him wallow. When he knew that I was withdrawing from him he put a last bit of effort into getting his brain into gear and he came to see Me for a little while, just visiting, he realised that he can crawl out of his apathy, talk and get things out of his system, realising things are worth crawling out of the darkness for, and he has now started to get a bit better. his daughter moving to Greece was a big part of his depression, and he felt that no one else cared for him as his daughter had.

I have managed to get him out of his house and spending time here with Me, pottering in the garden and teaching new slave some of the things he could do well, and he feels better by the time he's ready to leave. he is in Greece at the moment; I hope a month in the sunshine will make him feel better. I do know that while he is clambering on the rocks, he will fall in the water, he always does, he will get sunburned as I'm not there to nag him, but his daughter will make him feel better. As he had never been to an airport by himself before I knew he would get into trouble and I got a text to say he had got himself lost, I knew I should have put a badge on him saying 'I need help, please ask me.'

TEASE ME, PLEASE ME, WHIP ME, BEAT ME

I went to visit him and his family for two weeks, and bring him safely home, negotiating the dreaded airport so he didn't get lost. he had a mishap most days I was there, but winning Monopoly twice made his trip, it must have been a fluke, he only won the second time because I left the game early and all My blocking tactics went back to the bank for sale. he was a happy bunny though

My new garden slave is a masochist, I can do anything to him and he works all the harder for it. he came at a time when I needed some hard digging done. I needed foundations dug, ready for a summerhouse to be erected on. But firstly he made the garden tidy, mowed the lawn, weeded, sorted the pond out. he brought Me pots of plants and bedding plants, the garden was taking shape again...Ready for Me to disrupt matters by wanting to re-plan things.

I had ordered a summerhouse, which was to be delivered on a Wednesday. On Tuesday I took My mother shopping, a disastrous day, pelting with rain and we went to the wrong shops, the personal shopper we had wanted was not available and we got landed with an incompetent. We ended up coming home nearly as rich as when we started. I had left My phone in the car and found I had missed forty phone calls and they were still trying to get Me. Exasperated at missing a turning, and waiting at some lights, I had a feeling about a call coming through and took it; it was the chaps delivering My summerhouse. They were at My house and waiting instruction on where to put the pallet.

As garden slave was there I told them to put it on the driveway. I had wanted it near the house so cars could still park there, but when I had dropped by Mother at the station, the only thing that went right, she only waited five minutes for a train, I arrived home to find the bulky article had been deposited half on the drive and half on the pavement outside. Now where I live given half a chance, anyone with an eye for the main chance would take the opportunity, and bump into the offending article and sue Me. I was furious, fuming and spitting bricks!

Trying to round up people to move the bulk proved hard, the fact it was pelting with rain might have had something to do with it, but a phone call to garden slave, proved his devotion to Me. Ordered to come, he happily moved the heavy sections to the end of the garden by himself. I'm surprised he didn't give himself a heart attack or a hernia. My poor boy was a drowned rat by the time he finished, but a very happy drowned rat because he had done something that pleased Me immensely. The next day he moved them all again so they could be covered until they could be erected. he had a little help this time from My maid though.

It still hasn't been erected, as I'm waiting for a hot tub to be delivered and that seems to have had a few hitches on its journey to be delivered here, nothing seems to go to plan, but I'm sure it will be worth it when its all done.

Thoughts of erecting the summerhouse were dashed when I informed the planning people that I wanted to put a structure at the end of the garden. They miscalculated the square metres and made it into a house...I had to get a client to give Me a professional drawing to prove how small it is, lots of letters have passed and visits, all wasting time and now a postal strike has delayed the out coming decision. I'm hoping that by the time I get back from visiting slave in Greece all will be put up and ready for Me to use...fat chance...!!!!

Well I got back...and the summer house has been approved, but there is a glitch with the hot tub, do I put up the summer house and hope the tub will fit through the doors, or leave it lying on the grass getting wetter and wetter as each days pass, until the day the tub comes.

CHAPTER THIRTEEN

It has got to the stage in My life that I feel I need to help others learn, so I have taken on two apprentices. They want to learn more about working with clients. It is totally different than the scene way of dealing with things. Sooki has been in the lifestyle for many years, I met Her through the Munch and We have been friends for years and as My work has picked up. Two Domming became a good option. She came for a few sessions, which proved popular. She had fun learning, and as She dresses in a distinct fashion, She was a big hit. Things began to calm down though on the client front, and on the days She came, work dried up, it was like the kiss of death, She has an interest in TVs, that is where Her heart is, but She has found that things are not as straight forward as they seem, because a lot of TVs don't come to see professional Dommes, to learn how to make up and dress. They will phone and girly chat, but won't visit, they might make appointments, but they won't come, She got very disheartened by this, but is still persevering.

She thought She had got herself a little playmate, who She met at a local party, but discovered that, as with a lot of TVs they just want to play, i.e. have girly chats, be dressed, be preened and primped over, but not give anything back.

It is satisfying to start from scratch and view an end result, be it a client or slave, but when it is just someone out to get something for nothing there is a feeling of dissatisfaction at the end. I'm not on about monetary gain here, but the feeling of being taken for granted; that You are just there to provide what they want. She has discovered this, but I'm sure that the longer She is actively participating in My way of life; She will find a stable of TVs to preen over.

She has taken a fancy to My maid, and the attraction is mutual, they have a great time together. She dresses chrissy and the sparks fly and they play to their hearts content, with or without clients present. Sooki has found how useful chrissy is about the house doing odd jobs, but She is not too tolerant of the fact that even slaves have a busy life and can only do things when their normal life permits. My maid has a very hectic and fraught life, and My needs come first after her work, well she is My slave so she is a little torn between the preening she gets with Sooki and the satisfaction she gets from working with Me.

The other working with Me is Princess...Now Princess is special to Me. She is My Daughter. She comes in on two Domme sessions; She adds glamour to the scene and a lot of sexiness. She is six foot tall without heels, statuesque and has long blonde hair. She has as an expressive a face as Me, every emotion can be clearly seen and as She is still quite new to this, She has to mask some of the things She is thinking, but I can often look over at Her and know that the expression on Her face is masked on Mine. Not all Our clients know of the relationship between Us, but those that do, get a big kick from the fact.

My youngest Daughter and a bit of a rebel, though with a heart of gold. We had a tempestuous time when She was growing up, not the easiest time of Her life. She is hot headed and very stubborn, We had some spectacular augments, and neither of Us won, She takes after Her Mother a lot.

I get on well with My middle daughter but youngest and I can talk about anything, and I mean anything, some conversations even friends wouldn't talk about and I have made Her think more than once with the things I get up to. But I am growing old disgracefully and she's happy for Me, either that or I am a source of amusement for Her and Her friends, whatever, I don't care I'm happy.

She loves going to the parties and has a following of admirers. She loves dressing in My clothes, Basques are Her favourite. She loves the smooth feel of latex and will sidle up to Me just to stroke it, or if We are at a party. We have a friend who maids there, she always wears latex and loves people to stroke her and pet her and give her lots of compliments. Princess heads straight for her as soon as We arrive. her wife also wears it and they always look stunning, maid usually gets changed two or three times in the evening, so petting is always on the cards as not only Princess likes to sidle up and grope. Sooki, Princess and Myself are asked to play at these parties as is maid's Mistress and Wife. Luckily for the subs, We have different tastes and so We pair off and deal with the naughty boys or girls.

Subspace

One of these is a TV who I didn't know was new to the scene. I played with her after a boot licking session, I took her to a peak, she managed to get to subspace, and it was when I had looked after her, brought her down, that she told Me she had never done any of the things I had done to her before and so never reached subspace.

Being able to reach subspace is sometimes an achievement. The right frame of mind has to be reached. The thought of what is to come is usually enough to get into the right mindset.

Subspace is the body's own endorphins kicking in and sending your mind into a far better place where you feel soo good. If you hurt yourself badly the endorphins kick in to cope with the pain, adrenalin surges through the body and helps you feel better. In play your mind is on other things, so detached from the real world, caused by the pleasure and pain that is being given, so the drug like endorphins rush around the body and give you the out of body experience. A lot of energy is used during this time, and as the recipient can be exhausted after a session, aftercare is given.

If this is caused by a spanking session, once subspace has been reached it doesn't take hard blows to keep the person in this state, stroking, sensations on the area can keep the person there, but care needs to be taken when bringing the person down as they are drained of energy, uncoordinated in speech and mobility, not part of the real world for a while, so sitting them down and keeping them warm, feeding them chocolate or giving them orange juice is a good idea, and trying not to leave them, giving them a cuddle is good too.

she loved it. The next party, I played with her again, took her to subspace, but she was reacting too strongly and I brought her out of it and spent a long time bringing her down. Still in a state of euphoria she wanted to play again, greedy girl, but I wouldn't play. When I left I found she had found someone else to play with, her prerogative, but it displeased Me as anything could have happened to her, and I haven't played with her since.

When I play at Swamp, I have a school boy that I see to, he is into hard caning, he wears a cap and school uniform, he loves the slipper and plimsoll, but loves to see a nice patent leather pump on a female foot, he brings his own tawse, a leather one that gives a resounding slap. When he is slapped he emits a lovely smell of a good aftershave, and as his bottom gets hotter the smell gets stronger. When I have finished with his bottom he will pay homage to my patent shoes and kiss My hand as he says thank you. Then he will get Me a well-deserved drink and bring it to Me wherever I am, a good very respectful boy.

I advertise on a couple of sites that are for working girls. Quite a lot of the girls offer light Domination so I have offered to teach them the basics. One girl came to visit Me, she was a natural. We used My new garden slave to practice on; he was in his element as Sooki joined in as well. I found out she had been to parties and had something to do with the scene a few years ago. She was so confident I would happily work with her any day and if she took it up as a profession she would do well. She lay into slave and her aim was good once she was given pointers as to what not to hit.

A few others have enquired but as of now no one else has been to see Me. Though getting back from holiday I have had two enquiries, one from the site and one just out of the blue from someone close by who must have seen My web site. Also some one I met a few years ago at a party wants to set up in the same town as Me and wants to pick My brains. Now I'm not sure about that, but I don't think she will be competition, and if it means she will operate in a safe way, I will teach her.

I had an email one day from a man who researches escorts and puts them into a directory. He was doing a book on Dominatrix, had written a bit about Me and put so many stars against Me. Writing back to him, I asked him to meet with Me.

He came for a visit, not a session and rewrote and gave Me extra stars. He told Me he would tell Me when the book was out and send Me a copy, but the first I knew about it was some phone calls I got last week.... It's working on the advertising stakes at least, thank you.

Switches

There are many in the scene who are Domme but who switch for one reason or another, this can be because they enjoy the pain side of things or because they at some point in their lives need the release that being dominated can give them. It can work well in relationships, but can take a lot of working out.

I have a dear friend who is switch; She likes CP and a lot of BDSM aspects. She has recently started a relationship with another friend who is deeply submissive. Before this relationship She was in a D/S relationship, She was in the relationship to play, She was the submissive and loved all the things Her partner did to Her, as She loves pain, but she is Domme and needs to be in control as all Dommes need to be, it was a big upheaval when She left. She had serious health problems, and felt She needed more than just a D/S relationship. Her partner couldn't provide this, so She walked. It took a while for Her to get better. She still isn't 100% fit, but finding Her soul mate helped ease Her heartache. She has learnt how to play with a male submissive, before She had a female, She is teaching him how to administer CP on Her, he seems to be learning well, but its very hard for a true submissive to give pain. Being ordered to, eases the conflict a little, and knowing that he is pleasing Her helps the conflict even more.

I met Her when She was with Her D/S partner and it was in the early days of Me going to Swamp. It is a very sociable place and We get together and eat out together. He is totally Dom as I am totally Domme; We get on well and have many of the same ideals. We are both anti social to a certain extent, like Our own space, don't want to settle down with anyone, not just yet anyway, who knows things may change. We have set ideas, and like things our Own way.

He likes whips and is often on open ground in Bristol cracking His whip; He has a love of pinball machines and has a couple in His house. He went to a convention a little while ago, and so did My friend. They entered a competition, which My friend also entered, and low and behold She managed to do better than Him.

CHAPTER FOURTEEN

A couple of years after starting to work professionally, a man came to Me, he had lost his driving licence, so getting to Me was a feat. He said He was Dom but needed a release, so I played with Him. Things were not going right in His life, a divorce, a death in the family, work problems. He came back a few times and when He got His driving licence back the plans We had made came into fruition. We had talked of making a chamber from the room I was working from. He gave Me ideas He had done one before. The room colour and style was decided and I went on holiday, pissed off to the Caribbean on a cruise for two weeks. I had a great time and when I got back exhausted from the trip home I wasn't allowed to see the Chamber as it wasn't quite finished. I was happy catching up with My post until I was allowed upstairs.

The room was beautiful. The deep red of the walls and ceiling, the bed to become a four poster with drapes of deep red, the carpet to be cobalt, the bedspread and curtains to be black and gold, a mirror put opposite My cross, so clients can see themselves, walls covered on hooks to hold the many toys. Lights, old wrought iron ceiling and wall lights, medieval candle sticks, radiator and skirting painted black, and lots of other touches, I was a very happy Domme.
It has changed just a little since that time.

TEASE ME, PLEASE ME, WHIP ME, BEAT ME

At the same time, My bathroom had been made into a wet room, useful for many reasons, one being My infirmity, but also for play...........

This Dom has a knack of telling stories and embellishing on the truth, which doesn't really endear Him to Me, but I am long suffering, though drew the line at Him inferring that We were in a relationship when He was talking to others. I introduced Him to Munches and Swamp and He made friends, though My friends kept their distance as His highhanded manner came to the fore. He knew everything about everything, and tried to teach others, things He had never done Himself. He brought a new sub He had met on a site to Swamp. Boasted of the things We do there and the poor girl thought We didn't like Her as We kept our distance. she was not happy with how things were progressing in their relationship and a mutual friend kept telling her to get in touch with Me, she wouldn't because she had been told by her Dom how close We were! Eventually I made contact and Wwe became friends.

One day she asked Me to join a conversation on msn, I was horrified at the way he was talking to her. he was berating her, making this girl who had hardly any self-esteem, who was new to the Scene way of life, who had done her utmost to please him while she was with him, and now when she had broken away from him, was still having to put up with his unreasonable behaviour. I gave him a mouthful, which he didn't like and refused to speak to him from then onwards. I really don't think he knew what he had done wrong.

A Domme has Their slaves' best interest at heart. You nurture them, look after them, take care of them. If they need their self-esteem building up You do it. their job is to look after You and they have to be in the right frame of mind to do this. It's not a question of them being afraid of You or doing something because they feel they need to. Things are done for You because they respect You, adore You, love You, You have to earn this, not demand it.

he went on to restart his previous relationship, he has now moved away to be with her, she is not submissive but has learnt to do the things he likes and I believe they are very happy together.

My little friend on the other hand, met her Husband to be, online soon after, she fell for Him big time. she had got a bit of her confidence back and being with Him has made her into a girl who now knows what she wants and aims to get it, she can be a bossy little strumpet, but knows the limits she can go to, as her partner is her Dom. They are both great people and I am so happy to see My friend with the confidence she has at last got and is now getting all the things she deserves after having a crap life, she has worked hard all her life and just been shot down in flames at every turn, with little money she always tries to help others, so now its payback time, and she's getting her reward. I really wish her well.

When I was quite new at this, in the first eighteen months, I had a client that wouldn't show any emotion. I was to learn why a day or two after the session. I accepted the booking by e-mail, through a third party; a slave was dealing with some of My mail at the time. Things were hectic at the time, My computer was down and Daughter nagging Me to get it fixed, breathing fire at My back, a proper little Domme. She wanted to surf the net and chat to Her friends and was getting bad withdrawal symptoms, it was nearly as bad as Her PMS.

I had a houseful of people that couldn't solve the problems and I was getting more and more uptight. I was rushing around like a blue arsed fly trying to get Myself and things ready for My client and things were getting to Me. In need of a calming effect I had a quick slug of Bailies, now, I rarely drink so this must have been a fraught time for Me, drink and work don't mix, as I was to find out.

I got everyone out of the way and client arrives. I went through My usual routine; he was a tie and tease. he was a little unsavoury but nothing I couldn't cope with. Nowadays I will order them into the wet room and hose them down. he lay there just accepting, the worst sort, showing no emotion, and at the end just got up, dressed and ran out the door.

A bit perplexed I cleaned up and carried on with life after a job. A few days later I got an e mail from My slave, to say that the client had been in touch with him and had said the session had only gone ok, that I had stunk of gin and that he was disappointed that I hadn't been young slim and attractive, his words 'one mans meat is another mans................Not sure if the gin was referring to the Bailies or my Chanel perfume. Nowadays I chew gum and won't drink even if I'm taken to lunch before a session.

I have another client who has been to see Me a few times, that really can't show emotion, he is such hard work that I am exhausted at the end of a session. I try to get something out of him but can't get anything, not even a twitch of an eyelid. Here is where safe words really are needed, as I can't read when he has reached limits.

he takes all I give him then says red and I haven't felt or seen anything that might give Me a clue. he is the only client this has happened with luckily. he does enjoy the session, very much, he assures Me each time. he feels better than I do I'm sure, because I am just drained. It takes Me ages to get My mind sorted after him. I need to focus on something positive, think of something different, and if I don't have another client after him to perk Me up, I will be down for a few hours. The usual coffee and cigarette just don't work. I say I won't see him again, but always do.

Feelings of discontent

I discovered a yummy looking man while I was browsing the net, tall, interesting life and lifestyle. We got talking and as things got deeper I discovered that he wanted to be Dominated. This was not a problem for Me, I relished the thought and gave him some on line sessions, I thought things were going well and that Wwe were going to meet. Wwe had worked out a scenario, a bit extreme and done in public, then he told Me he had been to see someone else for his first experience. I hit the roof, how dare he. Well it was his life, let him live it. he hadn't enjoyed the strange things that had happened, he was unsure, things that I could have introduced him to and made them enjoyable. After I blew My top I wouldn't talk to him again. I left it about six months before I got in touch with him again, briefly, just to find out if he was happy and to see if he had pursued the life he had wanted. he had got no further in his quest to find someone or fulfil his fantasy, so I left the conversation quickly, gloating, but gave him some websites to join as a parting shot.

CHAPTER FIFTEEN

ANAL PLAY

A lot of vanilla people think that anal play is for gay men. They seem to ignore the fact that the anus is a sensitive sexual organ. Just stoking can give pleasurable feelings. Just as a lot of clients come to Me wanting strap on, not training, they seem to think they can go straight into it, not warm up or anything. If that floats their boat, ok, I will do that, take them in a brutal manner, but that isn't what they really want.

I always start a session of this sort with Me stroking and vibrating the anus with gloved hands. Warming them up, getting them sexually aroused. Very sensitive and open minded so that when it comes time for Me to enter them with a finger or thumb, the intrusion is welcomed doubly so. Fucking with fingers lets Me know how much they can take, so I can gauge how big a strap on I can use, but firstly I milk them. Stroking the prostate, mind sometimes its so deep that My finger won't reach and sometimes I'm trying in vain to find something that isn't there, as happened to Me not long ago.

I tried to find the walnut shaped lump to no avail, no matter how deep I probed, I thought it strange but wasn't going to say anything to him and when I explained to him what I was doing he told Me his little nut of pleasure was not there any more, he still enjoyed the anal though.

I consider My greatest accomplishment to be making a client cum through milking and seconds after making him cum. he couldn't walk for a fair while afterwards, his legs were made of jelly and his mind was away with the fairies. he had to take time to recover, laid on the bed, quivering and shaking. I try and strive for this if the client can relax enough, but sometimes they want it to happen too much. And it just won't happen. Sometimes I can get them to the point of coming but as it can feel like they need to empty their bladder they resist, some will say about this, then I can tell them that this is normal, the break to talk has stopped the feeling, there is no point in carrying on, the next time they know what to expect.

I use different sized vibraters, dildos and butt plugs, pump up, soft or hard, there is an enormous selection out there, as well as enormous toys to plug any size cavity. I am always finding new toys to buy. I dread to think how many thousands I have spent equipping My chamber, and as I have a love of all things connected with My work; I keep buying new toys and getting people to teach Me new things. I suppose I am jack of all the things I do, but master of none.

Though if I am told that I am crap at something I am doing, and I enjoy doing it, I would practice,

practice and practice some more till I got it right, but I have found that if I'm doing something I enjoy it seems to come naturally to Me. The act of fucking someone with a strap on is a powerful thing. They are under Your control, under You physically and mentally. Your body in contact with theirs, Your leg, Your stockings touching their bare flesh, your front pounding against their backside, Your hands gripping their hips as You pull them onto the strap on as you thrust deeper and harder, vicious or sensual.

I have been known to make some cum just by fucking them, reaching the all-important areas. Some will try to dictate how they want to be fucked; I have to decide, if I do it their way or My way. They are paying Me, but how do they want their value for money? Some want the control taken from them, taking what they are given. Some want it their way. No two clients are the same; I have to gauge what to give to who.

Fisting

A client came to see Me one day he enjoyed being fisted. Now this was something I had strived to do in the past but never succeeded. he knew this, and was willing to talk me through the procedure.

As anal play was nothing new to Me, I had the knowledge of warming up and giving sensations, so the next step of pushing fingers, then fist into the cavity was a natural progression. But what to do with fingers in that confined space, how to position them was the mystery. Pushing hard, harder than I had thought safe, then even harder, gripping My elbow, using My other hand to push My arm deeper and deeper, My fingers curling and finding a comfortable resting place, feeling the tightness on My wrist, the confined space gripping My fist. I flexed My fingers giving him some discomfort, but it's all about feeling full so I knew I wasn't doing anything wrong. I tapped My arm and then vibrated My arm, then he told Me to take My fist out. I did this, then put it straight back in again.

This was such a fantastic feeling, something I can't really explain, but I was flying as high as a kite, I'm not sure who was the highest though, he was as pleased as Me at what I had achieved, and to this day I get as much enjoyment as My clients, every time I do this.

I met another client through a website. he had a fetish for stockings and tights and anything that would fit up his bottom. he would dress in tights from head to toe, with a hole ready for his bum to be invaded. I would have a pile of stockings ready to be fed into his backside, a lot of lube and anything else I might like to introduce into the space I had created by My fist. Cans of fizzy drink were good. I push a stocking into the cavity and push it as far as it will go, then seek the second gate and push it into the opening. Now that is a very strange feeling, not as strange for Me as for My client I'm sure. I was not able to feed many into his rectum as he wished. his wish was to be able to poo them out over a period of time, but I did manage to fill his bum somewhat.

Covering a can with a stocking and lubing it, I was able to introduce it into his backside pushing it in as far as it would go.
 he was very satisfied with the results. Though he couldn't take a monster butt plug that I have in My possession. This butt plug is enormous, it tapers from a point to a width that is bigger than the largest fist, no one has yet been able to take it. Mind it has been close on a couple of occasions, with My ardent fisters. It is so large that putting a condom on it is a delicate business.

I have had a couple of aircraft steel butt plugs made for Me, polished to perfection, very heavy and beautiful in the craftsmanship. Another credit to Master Chopper.

When I first met Master Chopper He had a stall at Swamp, I looked at His stall and bought a few things, commissioned a few things and chatted with this amiable cuddly Dom. He had some ornamental nipple weights on His stall that I looked over but as I use fishing weights, was not really interested in. I later came in on a conversation He was having with another, and discovered that the nipple weights were in fact butt plugs....

In My opinion and that of the other Domme's, what He had produced was not really big enough to be butt plugs and I felt the shape was wrong, so I told Him the size and shape I needed, and after wincing, thinking I was joking with Him, trying to imagine such a huge instrument being inserted into anyone's anus. He questioned a few, and much to His amazement found what I said to be true. He made Me a huge butt plug, which I love using and then a smaller double ended one. He has also made Me several floggers. This Man is a craftsman and takes great pleasure in His work.

Fisting is a powerful experience. Many strive to be fisted and it can take a long time, maybe years to accomplish, for some it may never happen. It can take a long while of stretching and as I see clients irregularly it is not always possible to build them up to this stage unless they work at it at home.

I remember one client who said he had never been fisted before, but wanted it; he had not really played at home, so I was very surprised when I started to play with him. he was so relaxed that when I inserted one finger after teasing him analy, it quickly turned into two then three then four. I made sure that he was well lubed, and pushed My fingers up as far as I could and worked them well, stretching his anus, he didn't know how many I had in him, he was just enjoying the sensations. I then positioned My thumb, pushing harder, inching My fist further up him, working against the resistance, then with My fingers curled up snugly in his cavity, pushed harder and harder, slowly forcing My fist, My knuckles, the widest part of My hand, into the welcoming opening. It is a very powerful feeling to have Your hand up someone's bum, and the elation Wwe both felt was strong, though he wasn't surprised that My fist had managed to enter him totally, which leads Me to believe that he had practiced on himself quite a lot.

CHAPTER SIXTEEN

CBT Hard CBT

Tell me what You want to do to me.
What would you like to happen?
Anything You want to do!
Ok... That leaves Me with a lot of scope.
You can film it if You want.
Ok... even better.
As extreme as You want.
Ok let Me think about this then.

The day arrives and he gets sent upstairs, he has brought some frilly matching undies, a netting body suit, matching thong and stockings. They have pretty red hearts and red binding, he has managed to rip the suit putting it on, stupid boy but luckily it won't show as it's not a part that is going to be filmed, it is lower down, his intimate bits that will be the focus.

A bench, a block of wood, a hammer, nails, gloves, sharps box, antiseptic. All set... Camera at the ready, I am not expecting too much as this is a test shoot. Wwe are all new to this, so if Wwe get any footage I will be happy. Nails sterilized, gloves on, no need to cuff him, I just get him to hold the wood steady. A nail between fingers, hammer at the ready, I pull his ball sac out and hold it into place, the nail holding the skin out I then proceed to thump the nail into place. he does not flinch. I go to the other side, I am intent on what I'm doing, taking no notice of the outside influences, the camera going and others watching, I will get their reactions when I have finished.

By the time I have put eight nails into his ball sac it resembles a bat, he has not flinched, he is a real pain slut. I am determined to get some reaction from him, so I pull his cock out from his body, grab the foreskin and pull it over his knob, then clutching a nail, drag the skin as far as I can and then bang the nail in, through both thick layers, the other side needs to be the same so I grab the left side and repeat the procedure, still no reaction...Oh well, let him stay like that for a while.

I get some sharps and decide that I am going to pierce his nipples. I make a box shape around his right nipple and a star around his left. The star has six sharps, each point digging into the nipple; I like the star better as it's prettier and because it's also causing discomfort.

Next I want to do some lacing. So I place two sharps near his shoulder a couple of inches apart, then bringing them down towards his nipple, getting closer together the nearer I get to his nipple. When I have placed eight, I get some ribbon and lace it round the sharps, tying a bow as I reach the end. I am pleased with the end result, very pretty, red ribbon to match his hearts.

Lots of pictures are being taken and the photographer is a pretty shade of green by this time. But he is willing to continue. Stepping back to look at My handy work, I decide that the time has come to see how much pain he will take, as the nails didn't cause enough pain, perhaps if he is forced to wank that might give the desired effect. Using two fingers to rub his pinioned cock, forcing the skin to agitate against the nails, pulling the foreskin back and forth, stretching it even more, I watch, he's not being energetic enough so I tell him to go faster, the skin is being pulled right back, straining against the nails. The more pain it's giving him the bigger he gets, I had thought he was excited while I was nailing him but it doesn't take long before he is asking Me if he can come. I don't want him to come yet. So I say no, at which he eases up, not good…and I tell him so and he starts to rub with renewed vigour. This time I let him come.

The mess that is made looks worse than it is, a great bloody mess, but only a little blood has been shed, the cum is mixed with it, but the photographer thinks there is more than there really is and turns a brighter shade of green. Wwe haven't finished yet; the nails have to come out. There is more pain as I get the hammer and hook each one out and drop them in the sharps box, his manhood shrinking back to its normal shape, the droplets of blood being soaked up with antiseptic wipes and slave with a big grin on his face. Next the sharps are taken out and they bleed a little more, then lastly I undo the ribbon and pull the needles out. All swabbed and euphoric, slave is on a high, as I make sure he is comfortable another slave is tidying the mess and gore up.

I had another session with this slave a few months before. he had been plaguing Me to do some extreme stuff with him and Wwe had decided to do this outside. The day arrived, it was blowing a gale and pelting down with rain, the worst weather Wwe had had for a long time. Slave's work only allowed for this day. Wwe had postponed the week before because of the weather, which hadn't been as bad as this day. The good thing about the weather being bad was that as Wwe were playing at the bottom of the garden, under My huge apple tree, the children from next door would not be able to see what Wwe were doing. They had no excuse to play in the garden; if they had tried to come out they would have been blown off their feet and done a Mary Poppins.

Garden slave erected sheeting around the tree, shielding Uus from any eyes that might be prying from bedroom windows, blue sheets that crackled and billowed with the wind, trying to escape from the ties that fixed it to the branches.

Today Wwe are using string, the swing, a hose and water containers. Slave is told to strip, the cold weather not affecting him at all, but do I care if it is...no. Cuffing him, and securing him to a high branch, leaving his body exposed to the elements, allowing Me to abuse his nipples slapping and pinching. I grab hold of his tackle and tie rope around his cock and balls, sling the other end over a branch and attach it to the water container, then to make life interesting another is added. They are dangling from the branch, gently swaying with the breeze. slave is sent to turn the water on and the end of the pipe is put into the mouth of one container. Wwe stand watching as the water fills the first five gallon container, eyes moving from slaves straining body and extending bits, to the water gushing and bubbling into the fast filling pot. The first one filled, I move onto the second. This one doesn't take long and by this time slaves back is arching, his feet are off the floor, the containers are closer to the floor and Wwe are marvelling at the fact that his bits are still attached to his body. I think that as he is dangling he might like to swing a little bit, so I grab hold of a water container and tug it gently, not a lot happens so I tug a bit harder until I am swinging the buts to the ground, lifting him further off the ground and back, his manhood taking My full weight as well as that of the water containers.

Cutting him free, letting his bits breath I then prepare to let him sit on the swing. Then he is tethered to the swing, arms out of the way, his bits once again tied. A water container set between his legs and attached to his crown jewels. Nipple clamps put in place, let the fun begin...pulling on the clamps, I set him in motion, back and forth, his nipples elongating as I pull harder, and the swinging gets higher...until it meets resistance, he is held back by the string which is attached to the but which is weighted to the floor. Whichever way he goes, backwards or forwards he is stopped by this obstacle. The continual tugging on his teats pays off as first one slides from their anchorage point, then as I continue to tug on the remaining one, the last pops off. I don't think he has enjoyed the swing for long enough so I replace the clamps the other way round this time and swing him some more, till yet again they slide off.

Undoing the rope from the container, I get slave to bend a branch down low and attach said rope. I push slave on the swing to take up the slack, then let the branch go. I like that way of getting him swinging, but soon get bored

It's cold and wet, the wind blowing through the plastic sheeting, the hosepipe still running, mixing with the puddles that the rain has left, drips coming through the foliage. slave needs to be warmed up Methinks. I order him to lie on the ground, standing astride him I proceed to pee on him, My golden shower covering his torso, from his tied cock, the rope of which I'm tugging on the other end, to his face. Ears, nose, eyes and open mouth filled with the warm liquid. Telling him to swallow, then back to his cock...I tell him to wank as I tug on the rope at the same time as covering his bits and hand as he pulls himself off. The session has been such an exciting one for him and he asks to come after a short time, this I allow, and as the last drops of My piss hit his cock they mingle with his spurting cum. The cum shoots over his head and the remains, as the force dies down, mingles in puddles on his chest and belly with the fluid of My gift to him. he is untied, and he with the other slaves tidy up, as I go indoors to warm up.

This slave has more treats in store as I intend to brand his cock. I am going to use boiling water with a thin brand at first, then I am going to use the violet wand and burn him with this. I have already put My initials on the bum of new garden slave with the wand, he is very proud of them, but the penis is more delicate than an arse, so I'm looking forward to doing that as much as slave is. Wwe have also talked of tying him to the tow bar by his cock and dragging him along behind as I drive at various speeds, seeing how fast he can run.

I love to tie cocks with rope, they look very pretty, and pretty is my thing. I have blue soft rope, from a well-known DIY store, I get strange looks every time I go and buy meters and meters of the stuff. If they only knew. I tie the cord around the balls and wind it tightly till the balls are shiny. I then tap and scratch them giving differing sensations. I separate the balls with rope or leather separators. I hang weights from the rope and get the body to swing them back and forth then side to side. If they aren't energetic enough with the swinging I give them a word of encouragement, a threat of something nasty, soon gets them motivated. I grip the dangling, rope-covered sac between My finger and thumb and squeeze and tug, looking into their eyes the whole time, watching them wince and squirm. I have sheaths that cover the cock which are then tied tight and as they are teased to become erect the small sharp or long blunt nails dig into the skin. I so enjoy inflicting CBT, from tying their bits to the ceiling and swinging from the rope, to flogging, full force onto their erect members. I have one client that likes Me to use My barbed wire flogger, giving him blood blisters. All this done with a smile on My face and chuckles escaping from My throat as I do this. Leading to belly laughs as he jumps and yelps and writhes as the flogger gets harder and harder. Not all the CBT I do is hard, it doesn't take much to read a client, be able to take them to their limits and keep it there. Some enjoy the pain, and some can get to sub space.

I use sounds. Urethral stretchers, smearing lube over the eye of their cock, I insert the bar slowly into the opening. A small one to begin with, gently helping it slide down the length of the penis, easing it past any gates that are there. I can feel the sound as it goes down the penis, I let it go the whole length and even further, I let it go into the bladder, try to give as many sensations as I can, so I vibrate the sound and slide it up and down. I then use progressively bigger ones, stretching till they can take no more. Using sounds is a good way of scaring them.

I like to watch the expressions on their faces as they watch the sound going further and further inside them, I am feeling the entry of the sound as it goes down the pipe, feeling and gauging the depth of the metal, clients eyes widening as it reaches the bladder, the path of obstacles navigated, the sound turning at bends and negotiating gates, widening the path, sliding up and down in preparation for the next size up. Tapping and vibrating the sound to give different sensations, letting the sound escape up the urethra, by its own volition, for Me to push it back down again.

I have a favourite client that loves this, I saw him yesterday. I had just got back from a holiday and was jet lagged but just playing with him using sounds, hearing him moan and writhe and getting him to sub space perked Me up. he is so receptive, the perfect client. Letting them clear the tubes at the end of a session is a necessity. I always boil and sterilize the sounds and use anti bacterial wipes before, during and after play.

A parachute can be used to separate the balls from the cock, and weights can be hung from it. A cock flogger can be used on the cock or balls, or hands to slap or a pencil; anything can be used to give sensation and pain. I have a few clients that like to be well beaten on their genitals, with a normal flogger or My leather barbed wire cat o nine tails, made especially for Me, by My friend Master Chopper.

I have a client who gave Me a new toy the other day, a very simple clip with a bottle of water attached to it by string. This clamps onto the foreskin and the water bottle is tugging his skin down causing his cock to hide from the pain in his body cavity. I teased him by holding the bottle and tugging on the string, then letting the bottle drop with a thud to the floor, the clamp sliding along the foreskin as it chases the bottle to the floor. It was replaced immediately and I got him to swing his member with all attached. A clamp can also be used to squeeze the glans and treat in the same way as the foreskin.

I use an electrical box and put the bands around the penis, attach the wires and switch on the box. Remember this is a sound activated device, so client thinks he is safe when I move away from him, thinking that I have had enough of making his cock twitch. But always expect the unexpected with Me, because I will find a way to cause more pain while I am not near enough to touch the box.

Putting the box on the clients shoulder when I walk away, telling them not to drop it is a good trick. With the sensor turned up full, I make an unexpected noise, and set off the box, with a careful eye on the instrument in case it should fall when the involuntary jump caused by the shooting pains happens. If it should fall, the intensity is turned up more, and pulling their hips towards Me I will spank them, causing the box to work well with the slap of flesh on flesh resounding.

TEASE ME, PLEASE ME, WHIP ME, BEAT ME

I like to make a cast of cocks using wax, to cover the whole cock and balls. I don't care if they are covered in hair, its more fun pulling the wax off hairy appendages. Depending on clients pain threshold, I gauge the height to hold the candle as the drips can vary in heat, closer very hot, further up just hot, and to keep dripping on the same spot burns quite well. It takes a while to cover a cock and balls in wax, and to see the cast taking shape is exhilarating. Going back to patches missed, going over hot patches as they are cooling to make sure there is at least one very hot spot all the time, breaking off and covering the nipples. If the client is blindfold the sudden change in position will cause a good reaction, as it's unexpected.

Once a cock and balls are covered and it has cooled to a cast it is fun to wank the client, trying not to dislodge the cast too much and not let him come can be interesting and if the client has not shaved a very interesting sensation is added with the hairs being tugged.

Covering a cock and balls in pegs is fun, you can make some pretty patterns with these and using a whip to take the pegs off is excruciatingly painful if You do it one by one, and if You don't give the right flick to begin with and the peg doesn't come off, You need to keep trying, causing lots of lovely gyrations and moans. A smile...putting pegs from one side of the ball sack to the other, is very pretty, then pegs from the base of the cock to the tip, ending with a peg or two holding the foreskin in place, covering the glans. Ending with pegs under the balls leading to the anus, just to make sure the pleasure point is dulled.

Hot and cold water can be used to heat or cool instruments to apply to the body. Ice is good; though You have to be sure there are no sharp edges. Also ice can burn so if client can't have marks You have to be careful. If the body is blindfolded, they don't know which is being used adding to the fun. Hot or boiling water can be used to brand.

I use ice and wax with tie and tease. Lighting a candle so they hear the ignition then the smell of the candle, letting them know what is going to happen. Holding the ice in My hand and letting the drips splash onto client, blindfold, the body can't tell if the sensation they are being given is hot or cold. Then the wax is dripped on. Then using a pinwheel, running it over their body, going into the creases as well as over cock and nipples. Up and down legs and arms, using differing pressure, to give different sensations. I like to loosen the wax with a pinwheel; it can take quite a while to get it all loose and sometimes a lot of pressure.

I have a favourite slave that I like to use wax on, My sissy who loves to dress and loves to try new things. But as he hasn't much time to spare, time is limited, but putting him in My sling and having him helpless, knowing I can do whatever I want with him, but seeing his manhood encased in wax is an amazing sight.

Something else I like using is Chastity devices. I put My computer slave in one, an old metal device; he was to wear it all day at work. he couldn't get away with using it at home. I fitted it on him, teased him a little then got the key to unlock him, inserted said key and turned...nothing happened...to My amusement and I got a fit of the giggles. I kept trying to no avail, so he had a go, but he didn't have any luck. By this time I'm thinking yummy firemen, and voice this to him. he gave Me a look, which said he wouldn't be impressed if I took him to the fire station.

I found a safety pin in the dressing room, and took this to him, he fiddled about and couldn't get that to work, so I found a kirby grip. he played about some more, pulling his member at some strange angles to try and get it in the right position, Me giggling at his discomfort, at last managed to free himself. The visions of cute firemen and a squirming very embarrassed slave exasperated from sight, oh hell luck was not with Me that night. he took the device home and made the key fit, so he was able to use it the next day.

I have another slave, a client who wanted to be put in chastity; I'm not sure how he would hide it from his partner so I decided on a two-ring type. At the time I was putting My garden slave in the same one. Garden slave came back with the news that he kept falling out of it. I had told him to try squeezing his balls through the ring but he couldn't, they were too big, so I threatened to shred them and push them through. But the other slave came back with the same news. So even trying to stop the glans trying to escape with a band under the ridge couldn't stop the little trouser snakes escaping, back to the drawing board. Garden slave is in the gates of hell at the moment, but something has to be done to stop him having a little fiddle. Mind I do let him do that...just don't let him cum. I have just ordered a new device that involves trust...as its made of leather, I'm not sure how it works. It has arrived and I can't work out what a flap of leather is for, but I'm sure when I put it on him it will all fall into place. It does look rather big for a flaccid penis though. Made in leather with rings, that is made to measure, so I hope that works. I know garden slave won't abuse the trust there and have a quick wank without permission.

I put a slave in chastity through cyber. he bought the device after consultation with Me. When it arrived I got him to prepare in front of the web cam. To shave, now that is erotic to watch, as erotic as shaving the slave yourself, watching him pull his cock and balls about as the blade slides over the skin, the fresh skin being denuded...he had made the chastity device fit properly before the official caging, so it didn't take him long to encase himself and put the lock on. I took the number from the padlock and he was all set. I kept in touch with him every so often and it was a surprise to Me as to how his way of thinking about the opposite sex was changing. Before he would chat up the females, he was not in a relationship but did want to be. A short while into the experiment I stopped hearing from him. I thought he had given up and could not face Me. But after a couple of weeks he popped back online and the padlock was the same as the one Wwe had put on. he had been ill with the flu; his mother had been looking after him. I asked if she had seen the device, she hadn't but he had been so ill that he wouldn't have cared if she had. I got him to shave in front of Me, taking the cage off, then I let him wank in front of Me....but not cum, that was so hard for him and it took a long time for his erection to go down afterwards so he could go back to his chastity.

Sleep was difficult for him in the first few days, not being used to the obstruction when he turned, and as he was so horny, he used to wank 4 times a day. he used to get a lot of erections day and night, all of which now couldn't grow to fullness. he found that the way he talked to females had changed. he didn't need to chat them up any more, well he couldn't bed them now could he, if he did he would be breaking trust.

Wwe still kept in touch and he wrote a diary of his thoughts and feeling. he was not allowed to wank anymore and found he could shave without taking the cage off. The only down part of the experiment was that he emitted a lot of fluid and so he devised a little nappy of sorts. It didn't seem to show under his trousers, and the little chaffing he got, he was able to keep under control with cream. During this time, he found out that one of his fuck buddies was into the same things that he was and off came the cage. he didn't tell Me and when I found out I just told him he should have told Me. he put the cage back on and after a few days he came to see Me to take it off officially. Wwe had an enjoyable session and he went home happy to his new partner. Part of his story is on My website.

CHAPTER SEVENTEEN

My days

Every day for Me is different, that is the way I like it, I don't like uniformity and order, I have others around Me to create that order. I hate getting up early, but I'm not a night owl, I'm a complex character because if needs be I can be up and about early or stay up till the wee small hours.
I have learnt through experience to switch My phone off at night.

Sweet music playing, ooops it drags Me from the deepest depths, no not My alarm.

Grope for the phone, where the hell is it, got to get it quick, visions of Daughter stranded, needing Her Mum, bleary eyed can't see the number,

'Yea what's up?'
'Hello darling are you working tonight?'
'What the fuck, sod off............'

Punching the off button and switching the whole thing off, I'm wide-awake and cursing. No self-respecting submissive client would phone in the early hours of the morning, it was a rampant chap wanting his end away. Curses on him. I hope he gets the pox and his knob drops off.

Clients can phone from ten onwards, though if they have an appointment at ten they may phone to confirm at nine. I take on the day appointments as I very often see people who are down for the day on business. So I never know how My day is going to pan out. I might just spend the day talking to people who don't want an appointment; I sussed that early on and got Myself an 070 number. I get a few pence and the telecom company get many more... but at least I was getting something for chatting, My regular clients had My usual number.

I get money every month for this and it comes in handy as I spend a lot on advertising, but as I don't do My spread sheets every month I didn't notice that I was getting the cheques randomly until at least five months had passed, too late to get in touch with them. I can't remember who they are, typical Me lost the paperwork. They have quite a few hundred pounds extra in their pockets the b...s. I dread to think how many others they have done this to; they must be raking it in. Well no more with Me, the numbers have now been changed, but My Domination chats no longer get to talk to Me, as I won't do it for free. Bless them, they keep trying, but until I get a new number on a new phone they are left hanging or find someone else.

Time passes quickly as I spend a lot of time on the computer, answering e mails and chatting, between getting ready for clients, cleaning equipment and setting up, squeezing into rubber or choosing undies to put My sissies in. Texting slaves and running the house.

I don't watch much television, but that or the radio is always on in the background, and I have Nina Simone on, in a play session. You can guarantee that if I go shopping or have a meeting that the phone will go off, so I'm chatting to clients in the middle of Sainsbury, trying to merge into a stand so it absorbs My whispers. Rush the rest of My shopping to get home and get ready for a client that may or may not come, but such is life. Timewasters are a big part of this business and though they are annoying there is not a lot You can do about them. I don't take bookings made from withheld numbers seriously, I tell them to phone from a recognised number when they phone to confirm, not many do...

I take time off when I have My beautician come to visit Me. I know...too lazy to go to a salon...well that's Me all over. Anything for an easy life. She comes every fortnight and is here for hours, not only does she see Me but others come to join in the fun as well and laugh at each other as We undergo different treatments, slaves and friends and its like a party. She is so bubbly and vibrant, with her waxing equipment at the ready, just as I do with My clients, doesn't stop the mood. She is a real sadist with the wax, in fact she laughs at My grimaces, I don't resort to screams, but have been known to swear on occasion.

I also have a hairdresser who visits, Princesses best buddy, she knows that I love her work and has at long last got the confidence in it since a trip to Australia. Alas she is going back to live there next year, but while she has been away I have been seeing another friend of Princess who is also old garden slaves grand daughter, so she knows my lifestyle, which is handy.

I can't see Me giving up this lifestyle for a very long time and so long as My health permits I will keep working, because I love My work so much. I think it shows when I session with people as well. Well I hope it does.